SPECT

SINGLE-PHOTON EMISSION COMPUTED TOMOGRAPHY:

A PRIMER

SECOND EDITION

Robert J. English, CNMT
Research Technologist
Nuclear Medicine
Brigham and Women's Hospital
Boston, Massachusetts

Susan E. Brown, CNMT
Chief Technologist
Nuclear Medicine
New England Medical Center Hospitals
Boston, Massachusetts

Published by
The Society of Nuclear Medicine
136 Madison Avenue, New York, NY 10016-6784

The Society of Nuclear Medicine, Inc.
136 Madison Avenue, New York, NY 10016-6784

Library of Congress Cataloging in Publication Data

Main entry under title:
English, Robert J. (Robert Joseph), 1949–
    SPECT: single-photon emission computed tomography: a primer/
Robert J. English, Susan E. Brown.–2nd ed.
    p. cm.
    Includes bibliographical references.
    ISBN 0-932004-34-2: $15.00
    1. Tomography, Emission. [1. Tomography, Emission Computed.]
I. Brown, Susan E. (Susan Emery), 1949–
II. Title. III. Title.
Single-photon emission computed tomography.
    [DNLM: WN 160 E58s]
1. Tomography,
RC78.7.T62E54 1989
616.07'572–dc20   89-21808
                            CIP

Printing: 3 4 5 6 7 8   Year: 8 9 0 1 2 3 4 5

With thanks to

Carol A. English
and
David C. Brown

for their understanding and support

FOREWORD

This concise volume presents the essence of single-photon emission computed tomography in an understandable and practical manner. It is written for the professional nuclear medicine technologist and assumes the comprehension and experience expected of journey-men and women who are the mainstays of contemporary nuclear medicine practice.

The logic of the book is clear: history, principles, quality control, acquisition, processing, clinical utility, and applications of SPECT. The authors bring an experience born of working through the technology, using it in the clinical settings and of teaching it to others. SPECT is a here-and-now technique; this book tells you how to use it.

S. James Adelstein, M.D.
Boston, MA

PREFACE TO THE SECOND EDITION

By presenting in this edition procedures for routine and initial evaluation of a SPECT system as well as protocols for commonly imaged organ systems, we continue the principle objective stated in the first edition of this book: to assist nuclear medicine technologists in expanding their knowledge of nuclear medicine to include SPECT. The protocols and procedures are specifically presented here in a generic fashion to offer the greatest flexibility to both the novice and the more experienced practitioner.

We would like to acknowledge and express thanks to Marcia Boyd, CNMT, Chairman of the Publications Committee, Author Hall, CNMT, President of the Technologist Section, David Teisler, Eleanore Tapscott, Max Nigretto, and Martha Mirabito of the Central Office of the Society of Nuclear Medicine, and those past and present officers and committee members of the Technologist Section, The Society of Nuclear Medicine.

Robert J. English, CNMT
Susan E. Brown, CNMT

PREFACE TO THE FIRST EDITION

Our principal objective in writing this book is to assist nuclear medicine technologists in expanding their knowledge of nuclear medicine to include SPECT. The text of this primer is written with the assumption that the reader is proficient in most elements of nuclear medicine technology; therefore, the information is limited to data that will answer the basic questions of single-photon emission computed tomography. In order to apply this exciting dimension of nuclear medicine fully, the technologist is required to understand the operation of new equipment and comprehend the computer processing involved in the production of quality images. Learning the basic theory and quality control necessary to produce diagnostic images is the technologist's responsibility, since the integrity of the final product rests with the individual. Nuclear medicine technologists are obligated to continually update their competency of changing techniques and modalities.

It is unfortunate that as a new technique emerges and develops, the information related to it is often spread throughout a vast number of medical journals, lecture proceedings, and manufacturer's literature. We found this to be true with SPECT, an imaging modality that is finding an accepted place in the clinical setting. Our goal is to bring the basics of this material together in a manner that would answer the technologist's fundamental questions. We have designed this primer in a generic manner to be used as an extension of the manufacturer's operating manual. We are aware of the variety of SPECT devices available; we also acknowledge that a number of variances in acquisition and processing techniques are possible and not always addressed in this text. We concentrate on the rotating gamma camera because it is the most common type of SPECT system clinically available. While it is our hope that those not directly involved with SPECT will benefit from this text, its main purpose is to answer the technologist's usual "Why?" when following an equipment procedure manual.

This book is not meant to be an exhaustive source of data, but rather a study guide of the technology and application of SPECT. A glossary is included which contains some of the terminology relevant to the specialty, and reading lists are provided at the end of each chapter to direct the reader to more comprehensive text on specific subjects. Finally, study questions are available for your use.

We wish to acknowledge and express thanks to B. Leonard Holman, M.D., Vincent Cherico, CNMT, Chairmen of the Publications Committees, James Wirrell, CNMT, President of the Technologist Section, Laura Kosden of the Central Office of the Society of Nuclear Medicine, and those past and present officers and committee members of the Technologist Section, The Society of Nuclear Medicine.

Robert J. English, CNMT
Susan E. Brown, CNMT

ACKNOWLEDGMENTS

We would like to thank the following individuals for their assistance in the preparation of this book:

B. David Collier, M.D.
Medical College of Wisconsin
Department of Radiology
Milwaukee County
Medical Complex
Milwaukee, WI

Angelika Haag, NMT
Division of Nuclear Medicine
University of Munich
Munich, West Germany

Paul C. Kahn, M.D.
Tufts University School of
Medicine
Division of Nuclear Medicine
New England Medical Center
Hospitals
Boston, MA

Carl-Martin Kirsch, M.D.
Division of Nuclear Medicine
University of Munich
Munich, West Germany

B. Leonard Holman, M.D.
Harvard Medical School
Division of Nuclear Medicine
Brigham and Women's Hospital
Boston, MA

Charles W. Piez, M.D.
Erlanger Medical Center
Department of Radiology
Chattanooga, TN

Stephen C. Moore, Ph.D.
Harvard Medical School
Department of Radiology
Brigham and Women's Hospital
Boston, MA

Sabah S. Tu'meh, M.D.
Harvard Medical School
Division of Nuclear Medicine
Brigham and Women's Hospital
Boston, MA

Robert Zimmerman, M.S.
Harvard Medical School
Joint Program in
Nuclear Medicine
Boston, MA

CONTENTS

1 INTRODUCTION

HISTORICAL PERSPECTIVE

The roots of single-photon emission computed tomography (SPECT) date back to 1917 with the publication of a paper by the Austrian mathematician J. Radon. In this publication, Radon stated that a two- or three-dimensional object can be reconstructed from the infinite set of all its projections. In 1922, several radiologists working independently devised the method for moving an x-ray tube over a patient, while the film beneath the patient was moved in the opposite direction. This method blurred all but one sharply focused plane of the target. This linear tomographic x-ray technique would remain the traditional method of obtaining three-dimensional information until the advent of computed tomography (CT).

The work of these pioneer radiologists progressed (unaware of Radon's publication) until 1961, when Oldendorf developed a crude apparatus for gamma ray transmission imaging with an ^{131}I source. In 1963, Kuhl and Edwards developed an emission tomography system, and in 1966, a transmission system using ^{211}Am with oscilloscope-camera systems for data storage. Although the mathematical and physical concepts of image reconstruction were independently conceived in the early part of this century, the practical applications would have to wait until the advent of the modern computer.

Radon's technique of image reconstruction was repeatedly

"rediscovered" by mathematicians, radioastronomers, electron microscopists, medical physicists, and radiologists. After remaining dormant for years, the techniques of image reconstruction were first put into practical use in the field of radioastronomy by Bracewell (1956) for the purpose of identifying regions of the sun that emit microwave radiation. In the years that followed, image reconstruction was used in electron microscopy in an effort to reconstruct molecular structure from a series of transmission micrograms taken at various angles.

In medical radiography, the x-ray CT scanner introduced by Hounsfield in 1973, had a tremendous impact on diagnostic medicine. This event, however, was preceded by the emission tomographic radionuclide brain-imaging work performed by Kuhl and Edwards in 1963. In 1967, Hal Anger implemented the concept of the rotating gamma camera by rotating the patient at predefined angles in front of the detector. For the next 10 years, while x-ray CT exploded in the marketplace, several pioneering nuclear medicine physicians and scientists (Kuhl, Budinger, Keyes, Jaszczak, and others) worked relentlessly in developing SPECT. The success of their efforts is now clearly demonstrated not only by the commercial enthusiasm seen in the marketplace, but in the clinical excitement exhibited throughout the literature as well.

WHY SPECT?

The recent emergence of SPECT as a permanent imaging modality in nuclear medicine carries with it the question, "What are the advantages?" To the person working routinely with SPECT, this question is often answered with the question, "How do you do without it?" When the clinician or technologist first encounters SPECT, it may appear to be a technologic nightmare, consisting of such strange terms as projections, ramp, partial volume effect, voxels, and frequency cutoff. SPECT is simply one step further in the ability of nuclear medicine to improve diagnostic accuracy, not unlike the transition from the rectilinear scanner to the gamma camera.

The most apparent advantage of SPECT is simply its ability to remove the superimposition encountered in two-dimensional imaging. This might be best demonstrated by the problems found in imaging the ^{201}Tl distribution in the left ventricle. Patients with a large left lobe of the liver or demonstrating substantial lung uptake often pose a problem when the clinician tries to locate areas of decreased ^{201}Tl perfusion. Doubt as to the distribution of this radionuclide is largely removed by slicing through the long axis of the left ventricle. The decreased biologic and geometric constraints of ^{201}Tl have led to a modest improvement in the accuracy of interpretation. Another important factor in the ability of SPECT to section an organ tomographically is its potential of quantitative tracer measurements. This methodology, although still in an early investigational stage, may permit the measurement of physiologic functions that have eluded the nuclear medicine specialty in the past.

An illustration of the ability of nuclear medicine to demonstrate physiologic as opposed to morphologic changes, as well as the ability of SPECT to enhance it, has been presented by Holman and Hill (1984) in the diagnosis of cerebrovascular disease with ^{123}I-labeled amines. Within hours after the onset of stroke symptoms, SPECT images delineate the areas of abnormality, while CT images take up to 4 days to document the involved area. Functional imaging is not limited to the brain. Several investigators are producing work in the area of quantitative ^{201}Tl distribution in the left ventricle of the heart.

Keyes (1982) made the following observation concerning SPECT:

It is a technique that will enhance many of the things that we do in nuclear medicine but it certainly is not going to revolutionize the field in the same way that x-ray CT has changed the field of radiography. What we can hope for is a small but measurable improvement in diagnostic performance in many conventional imaging procedures, and the addition of depth to many of our developing attempts to provide functional data for the clinician. The ability to visualize radiopharmaceutical distributions in the body in three dimensions, the ability to quantify these dimensional relationships, and finally the ability to extract true quantitative values noninvasively from structures deep within the body should provide significant improvements in the way we practice nuclear medicine.

INSTRUMENTATION

The mathematical concept of image reconstruction has been around for a number of years, but the key to the success of its applications in CT, SPECT, PET, and MRI has been the development of the modern computer. The calculations required for image reconstruction are so complex that without the computer today's routine studies would be an impossibility. While the computer/gamma camera marriage has recently become commonplace in the clinical nuclear medicine setting, the computer interface has been the backbone of SPECT since its inception.

During the past two decades, SPECT has evolved from Kuhl and Edwards's "image separation radioisotope scanning" (1963) to today's commercially available rotating gamma camera systems. Nuclear medicine has seen SPECT instrumentation develop in the form of Keyes' humongotron, Stokely's dynamic computer-assisted tomography (DCAT), the Aberdeen section scanner, seven-pinhole collimators, rotating slant-hole collimators, Fresnal zone plates, and Stoddard's multidetector system, presenting a vast array of unique tomographic techniques. Each of these early concepts contributed to the understanding and development of the present state-of-the-art technology. Although each manufacturer markets a scintillation camera system with its own unique SPECT characteristics, all function within a generic framework.

This basic framework consists of a collimated detector system capable of acquiring data at varying degrees within a 360° radius, a method of converting analog signals to digital, and a computer system for manipulating, reconstructing, displaying, and storing data. Most commercial systems are rotating gamma cameras and, although peripherals, electronics, and software may be unique for each manufacturer, all operate from the same basic principle.

As with all nuclear medicine equipment, the system as a whole is very much dependent on each individual component. The finest intrinsic resolution can be negated with a poor choice of collimator. Even with the finest resolution, highest possible statistics, and ideal uniformity, the final image may be of poor diagnostic value if the patient moves during acquisition.

SINGLE-PHOTON RADIOPHARMACEUTICALS

An important plus for SPECT—although some may argue that it is a limitation—is its utilization of single-photon emitting radionuclides. While these radiopharmaceuticals are difficult to engineer biochemically, a large number are used routinely; they are comparatively inexpensive and accessible to the entire nuclear medicine community. It is this interrelationship that makes SPECT a useful diagnostic tool for all nuclear medicine services, and not restricted to research centers.

Radionuclide imaging has the potential to quantitate radiopharmaceutical uptake in regions of the body and thereby deduce function. With planar imaging, this capability has been limited by the distortion caused by attenuation and contributing count statistics from underlying and overlaying organs. Technologic advancements in SPECT bring nuclear medicine one step further to overcoming these restrictions. This may add a new value to our current inventory of single-photon radiopharmaceuticals and possibly pave the way for the introduction of new compounds. Until recently, the methodology of functional imaging had been dominated by positron-emission tomography (PET). However, the need for an on-site cyclotron and radiochemical/radiopharmaceutical support has limited PET to very few clinical sites. Techniques that use single-photon radiopharmaceuticals and that are free of high-technology costs could have widespread clinical value.

As an example, until recently the noninvasive measurement of regional blood flow has been limited to expensive and specialized instrumentation. The use of SPECT and the radiolabeled amines has permitted the detection of altered perfusion in neurologic diseases, such as cerebral infarction and epilepsy. The physiologic information derived from SPECT imaging of ^{123}I iodoamphetamine complements the anatomic and morphologic information provided by transmission CT. Planar imaging of radiolabeled amines has generated some interest, but the data achieved from SPECT imaging have demonstrated a greater increase in clinical information, made possible by a combination of both a new radiopharmaceutical and an imaging modality.

Thallium-201 myocardial scintigraphy has emerged as a routine test in the evaluation and management of patients with coronary artery disease. Although SPECT has added new dimensions and accuracy to this examination, it still faces the physical constraints of poor imaging photons. Technetium-99m is an ideal radionuclide for Anger camera scintigraphy because of its availability, short half-life, and 140-keV gamma energy.

Recently Holman and Jones (1984) described a new class of technetium complexes—the hexakis (alkylisonitrile) technetium (I) cations—which show excellent myocardial uptake. The substantially higher photon yield of this ^{99m}Tc compound permits faster imaging times in a SPECT mode; furthermore, the energy resolution of the ^{99m}Tc photopeak may produce an improved image.

Prospects for the further development of several agents currently being investigated have been improved because of SPECT, and a number of established clinical procedures have developed an increased potential with the added application of the SPECT modality. For example, the extent of metastatic disease in the liver is often better defined with SPECT than with planar imaging. Deep-seated or small hemangiomas may remain undetected with conventional planar imaging of technetium-labeled erythrocytes but can be observed clearly when overlying activity is separated with SPECT. Regions of ^{67}Ga uptake in the area of the mediastinum are better visualized when the activity of the sternum and vertebral column is removed. Temporomandibular joint abnormalities are easily demonstrated when the ratios of each joint are unaffected by structural superimposition. These complementary roles of SPECT all contribute to an increased accuracy in nuclear medicine.

THE ROLE OF THE
NUCLEAR MEDICINE TECHNOLOGIST

Unlike any other aspect of nuclear medicine, the computer has placed the requirement for excellence in imaging and diagnostic integrity with the technologist. SPECT increases this responsibility by making the final image, a function from quality control to image processing, completely user-dependent. Improper methods of uniformity correction, or center-of-rotation alignment, may place "hot" or "cold" artifacts in the image. On the other hand, excessive or incorrect filtering or attenuation correction may blur true abnormalities. Finally, improper display methods could place a defect in the incorrect part of the organ being evaluated.

SPECT places increased responsibility on the technologist for technical excellence. Nuclear medicine imaging techniques have come a long way from the simple calculation of information density on a rectilinear scanner. Today's technologist must be familiar with these equipment changes and cognizant of current imaging techniques.

SUGGESTED READINGS

1. Anger HO. Tomographic gamma ray scanner with simultaneous read-out of several planes. In: Gottschalk A, Bech RN, eds. *Fundamental Problems in Scanning.* Springfield, IL: Charles C Thomas, 1968:195-211.

2. Brooks RA, Di Chiro G. Principles of computer assisted tomography (CAT) in radiographic and radioisotopic imaging. *Phys Med Biol* 1976;5:689-732.

3. Gordon R, Herman GT, Johnson SA. Image reconstruction from projections. *Sci Am* 1975;233:(4)56-68.

4. Holman BL, Hill TC. Functional imaging of the brain with SPECT. *Appl Radiol* 1984;13(6):21-7.

5. Holman BL, Jones AG, James J, et al. A new Tc-99m-labeled myocardial imaging agent, Hexakis(t-Butylisonitrile)-Technetium(1) [Tc-99m TBI]: Initial experience in the human. *J Nucl Med* 1984;25:1350-55.

6. Keyes JW. Perspectives on tomography. *J Nucl Med* 1982;23:633-40.

7. Kuhl DE, Edwards ED. Image separation isotope scanning. *Radiology* 1963;80:653-62.

2 IMAGE RECONSTRUCTION

Reconstruction of a third plane from a series of two-dimensional images has undergone a transformation from the simple and crude to the complex but elegant. Each computer technique, or algorithm, used in CT constitutes a unique approach to image reconstruction that has evolved from a single basic concept called backprojection. Although it is not within the scope of this text to describe all these techniques, a discussion of some fundamentals is warranted.

BACKPROJECTION

The backprojection technique is a crude but simple method of obtaining an approximate reconstruction from multiple projections. Because of its simplicity, backprojection may be used graphically, photographically, or electronically. This was the technique used by Kuhl in the early 1960s to produce the first emission tomograms and, although not used today, backprojection provides a foundation for understanding the methods and problems of present-day reconstruction techniques.

The backprojection is a composite of all the ray sums of multi-angled, two-dimensional views, such as those that may be acquired with a scintillation detector. When projected onto an image field (such as film, paper, or computer matrix), the overlap, a result of the ray sums projected at their respective angles, represents a cross section or a new plane of the original source. The concept of a ray sum might be best described if we consider a point source acquired onto a 5 × 5 image matrix at pixel location 3,3. For the sake of simplicity, this point source could be given a value of 1, occupying pixel 3,3 on a single planar image. If this one projection is backprojected onto a new matrix, the value of the point source (in this case 1) would be placed in all the pixels representative of the angle of data acquisition. If the planar image is an anterior projection, a value of 1 would occupy all the pixels in column 3 (*y* direction) of the backprojection matrix. An image collected in the right lateral projection would place a value of 1 in all the pixels of row 3 (*x* direction); the result would be the addition of the values in pixel 3,3 that would yield an additive value of 2 at this one point, where column 3 and row 3 cross. The assignment of the source value to all the pixels along the path of acquisition converts this discrete point to a ray, or the ray sum. A simplistic digital example of backprojection might take the following form:

Planar Projection	Anterior Back-projection		Lateral Back-projection		Final Back-projection
00000	00100		00000		00100
00000	00100		00000		00100
00100 ⟶	00100	+	11111 ⟶		11211
00000	00100		00000		00100
00000	00100		00000		00100

The backprojection technique is often referred to as a "brute force" attack on image reconstruction because it collects the source as a complete sum and projects it back, as that sum, to each imaging area (pixel) along that path of the acquired angle (Fig. 2-1A). A point source collected and backprojected in this manner would build up an increased density where all the ray sums crossed and would present a representation of the point source from a new perspective (Fig. 2-1B).

To better appreciate the localizing ability of backprojection, consider four independent sources, suspended within the 360° field-of-view of a rotating gamma camera (Fig. 2-2A). A standard

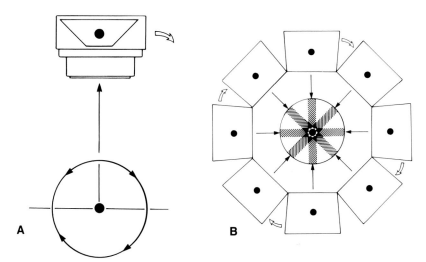

FIG. 2-1. (**A**) Acquisition of source into first projection bin, and (**B**) back-projected distribution of source into all picture elements along acquired projection's representative angle. Cross section of source distribution is represented by the criss-cross of backprojected ray sums.

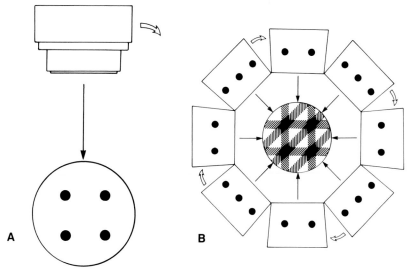

FIG. 2-2. (**A**) Vertex view of four point sources in a gamma camera's rotational field of view, and (**B**) backprojection of planar projections with resultant criss-cross indicative of transaxial point-source distribution.

anterior planar view would display the distance between the source in that plane, but not the depth, and a lateral view would present the depth but would provide no indication of the spatial separation seen anteriorly. It becomes clear that the best plane of reference is that of Figure 2-2A, which is impossible to achieve with standard planar imaging, with the possible exception of the vertex view.

With the backprojection technique, a transaxial view is achieved by acquiring predefined angulated views, then projecting each view at the angle of data acquisition onto a matrix as a ray. The acquired point sources shown in Figure 2-2A will be projected as rays that cross each other at the location of the original source(s) (Fig. 2-2B). The "star" effect surrounding the projected images is attributed to the complete projection of the point as a ray. In our 5 × 5 matrix example, the 1 values radiating from the crossover point, or 2 value, are typical of the star artifact. These artifacts, not present in the original source, will significantly degrade the quality of a more complex image such as the human head. A more elegant technique, such as those using filters, will present the sources as distinct points.

Backprojection in this raw form is not used today but does provide some historic background to the problems encountered in reconstructing an additional image plane and also supplies a fundamental insight to the understanding of the analytic methods of image reconstruction. A mathematical model of backprojection is described in Appendix D.

ANALYTIC RECONSTRUCTION TECHNIQUES

Filtered (Convoluted) Backprojection

The most common method for removing the star artifact is the introduction of a filter to each individual projection. Consider again the backprojection of a single point source and the density histogram applied to the ray (Fig. 2-3A). Filtering may be accomplished by the introduction of small negative values to each side of the peak in the ray histogram (Fig. 2-3B). When these filtered views are reprojected, the negative values will in effect cancel or erase all but the highest-density portion of the ray sum (Figs.

2-3C,D). If the filter is of an ideal design, and if enough projections are acquired, the cancellation effect might be perfect and result in a close representation of the original source. A multitude of sophisticated mathematical filters exist, but this basic concept of filtered (convoluted) backprojection is used in most commercial software packages. The classic commercial filter package avail-

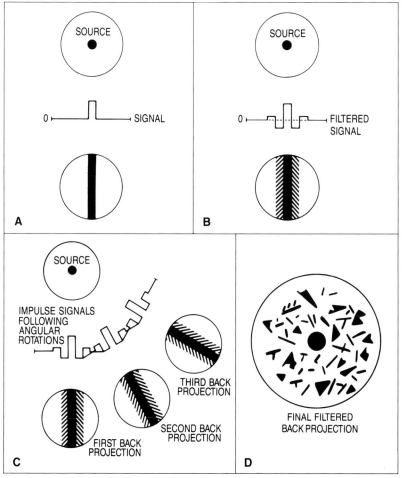

FIG. 2-3. (**A**) Unfiltered backprojection of point source, with resultant ray-sum and density histogram. Negative value (filter) applied to (**B**) first density profile and (**C**) each of the following projections. (**D**) Final filtered backprojection of point source with suppression of "star" artifact.

able today is the ramp filter, with a window cutoff. Filters and windows are described in more detail in Chapter 4 and a mathematical approach to filtered backprojection is outlined in Appendix E.

Two-Dimensional Fourier Reconstruction

In backprojection a "brute force" technique was used to reconstruct an image. It simply applied all mathematical sums of all pixels along a predesignated path. A straightforward solution of the mathematical equations of reconstruction can be achieved by two-dimensional Fourier reconstruction. It might be helpful in understanding the concept of Fourier transformation by first accepting that data, or counts per pixel, can be portrayed in both real space (the image), or in frequency space (a series of sinusoidal curves or waveforms). If one considers that pixels are continuous but bounded repetitions, or frequencies with a distinctive separation, and the counts in a pixel are labeled as amplitude, a basic pixel distribution in a planar projection might look like Figure 2-4A in real space and like Figure 2-4B in Fourier space. The curve plotted in Figure 2-4B provides an assessment of the pixel distribution makeup, with a series of curves that can be easily stated in mathematical terms. When the Fourier transform is interpolated into a rectangular array (Fig. 2-4C), the image is easily reconstructed by simply taking the inverse Fourier transform of the array (Fig. 2-4D).

The elegance of the Fourier transform technique lies in its straightforward analytic approach; that is, if the mathematical expression for a given shape is known, the necessary sine and cosine waves to synthesize that shape can be determined by performing the Fourier transform on that expression. These data can then be projected and the process repeated with each new angular sample. The simple application of an inverse Fourier transform technique can convert the reconstructed data into real space.

Fourier transformation attempts a direct solution to equating observed values with transverse distribution. Although mathematically "clean" and capable of yielding excellent reconstructions, this method is limited by spatial resolution but is not necessarily restricted because of the limited resolution of nuclear medicine im-

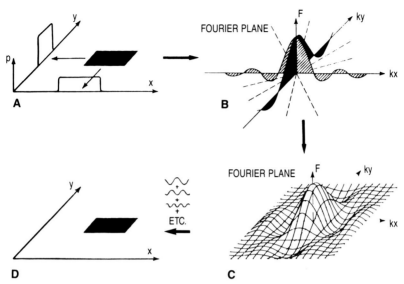

FIG. 2-4. Two-dimensional Fourier reconstruction. (**A**) Two right-angled projections of a rectangular object. (**B**) Fourier transform of the two projections, and (**C**) interpolation into rectangular array. (**D**) The image is reconstructed by taking the inverse two-dimensional transform of the Fourier coefficients. (Courtesy of Brooks RA, DiChiro G, *Phys Med Biol* 1976;21:689-732.)

aging devices. However, the long acquisition times and limited computer capacity of SPECT necessitate the use of a faster, filtered backprojection technique in most commercial devices. Further mathematical details of Fourier transformation are given in Appendix F.

Convolution filtering is generally used for speed and simplicity. Fourier filtering is potentially faster, but implementation difficulties have prevented routine use of this technique. The main problem is that the Fourier transform method cannot be applied until all projections have been acquired, whereas filtered backprojection can be applied to projections one at a time. This situation will probably remain in effect as long as collection times remain greater than 10 sec per projection.

Readers seeking a detailed explanation of the physics and mathematics of SPECT may refer to Nahmias's chapter, "Understanding Convolution Back Projection" and to Todd-Pokropek's chapter, "The Mathematics and Physics of Emission Computed Tomography (ECT)" as described in the reading list.

ITERATIVE METHODS OF RECONSTRUCTION

Backprojection reconstruction techniques provided the first steps to image reconstruction but demonstrated poor, artifact-ridden images. The first generation of algorithms used for medical applications were the iterative algorithms. To appreciate the concepts of the iterative methods of reconstruction, consider the acquisition of counts from a source stored in a 2 × 2 matrix. The true distribution might appear in cross section as follows:

4	3
2	5

Each number represents the cross-sectional counts per unit of area. The distribution of counts (ignoring photon attenuation) seen on the planar views would have the following appearance:

Anterior

	6	8	
7	4	3	7
7	2	5	7
	6	8	

Posterior

The problem arises when one considers that there is no precise prior knowledge of the true count distribution within the matrix. With only the static views to work with, an educated guess has to be made as to the count location. The reconstruction process begins with the following situation:

```
          6        8
      ┌──────────────┐
  7   │  ?        ?  │   7
      │              │
  7   │  ?        ?  │   7
      └──────────────┘
          6        8
```

and might possibly be reconstructed as

```
          6        8
      ┌──────────────┐
  7   │  3        4  │   7
      │              │
  7   │  3        4  │   7
      └──────────────┘
          6        8
```

This solution may be mathematically correct but when compared with the original source distribution, it is wrong. If, however, the number of views were to be increased to include obliques, the number of possible solutions would be considerably reduced:

```
  9       6        8       5
      ┌──────────────┐
  7   │  4        3  │   7
      │              │
  7   │  2        5  │   7
      └──────────────┘
  5       6        8       9
```

These additional projections have, in a very simplistic example, displayed only one solution, substantiating the theory that an infinite number of projections will approach reality. This example is only a 2 × 2 matrix, with a total of four pixels. Consider the situation of iterating through sixty-four projected 64 × 64 reconstruction matrices. It becomes obvious that a computer is a necessity.

A number of iterative reconstruction algorithms have been developed, including the algebraic reconstruction technique (ART), the iterative least-squares technique (ILST), and the simultaneous iterative reconstruction technique (SIRT). Basically, these iterative methods produce a series of approximations beginning with the setting of all values equal to 1 or a simple backprojection or any other reasonable first guess. This result is then projected to yield ray sums. These first-guess ray sums are then compared with measured ray sums, and a correction factor derived from these comparisons. The ray corrections are backprojected and added (or multiplied) to the current solution. This entire process, starting with the projected ray sums, is repeated a number of times until an approximate solution within some acceptable criterion of the true result is reached. The order and updating techniques of the corrections are what distinguishes the algorithms.

PHOTON ATTENUATION

The exponential attenuation of photons by the patient's body makes it difficult to obtain accurate quantitative information about radiotracer uptake in SPECT. As illustrated in Figure 2-5, even the 511-keV photons used in PET have less than a 40% chance of traversing 10 cm H_2O without being absorbed or scattered. However, in positron tomography, the simultaneous detection of two back-to-back photons makes it much easier to correct for this attenuation with some assumptions concerning measurements of the extent of attenuating material. In SPECT imaging, the photons are usually of lower energy, making them more strongly attenuated by the same material.

Perhaps a more serious problem for SPECT is the measurement ambiguity that makes it difficult to correct projections before reconstruction. One hypothetical projection ray is shown in Figure 2-6. It is easy to see that the same measurement (P) could be obtained by imaging a strong source (A) attenuated by length D_a,

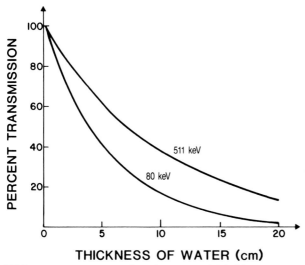

FIG. 2-5. Percentage of positron and 80-keV gamma photons transmitted through water. (Courtesy of Moore SC, *Computed Emission Tomography* New York: Oxford University Press.)

or imaging a weaker source (B) attenuated by a shorter distance D_b. Thus, in SPECT, the measurement process "mixes" the activity distribution with the distribution of attenuating material.

Figure 2-7 is a uniform "flood" phantom reconstructed without any attempt to compensate for attenuation. The superimposed plot of activity concentration along a horizontal line throughout the middle of the cylindrical source demonstrates the pronounced decrease in the middle, which is characteristic of attenuation.

Several first-order correction methods have been proposed to compensate for attenuation. Such methods generally do not remove the measurement ambiguity; nevertheless, for uniformly attenuating cross sections and fairly uniform activity distributions, they may work adequately. With these methods, the attenuation correction factors can either be applied to the raw data before reconstruction (precorrection) or to the reconstruction image (postcorrection).

The methods of correcting for photon attenuation discussed in Appendix G are a sample of the ongoing efforts to minimize the constraints caused by attenuation in SPECT. Perhaps no other

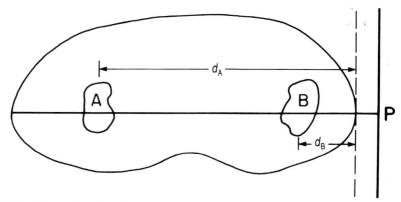

FIG. 2-6. Ambiguity of projection measurements in SPECT. Strong source A, attenuated by distance d_A, can yield the same projection ray-sum measurement P, as would a weaker source B, attenuated by distance d_B. (Courtesy of Moore SC, *Computed Emission Tomography* New York: Oxford University Press.)

single factor restricts the ability to achieve absolute quantitation in nuclear medicine as attenuation. The daily practice of SPECT will require the user to make use of or ignore the commercially available attenuation correction algorithms. The proper application of some of these techniques, particularly in homogeneous distributions such as the liver, will add to the overall content of the final image. The user must be aware, however, that cross sections of nonuniform attenuating tissue, as is found in the chest, may prevent proper attenuation correction with any of the commercially available first-order techniques. Again, as with data manipulation in general, the applications and advantages of attenuation correction depend on the needs and acceptability of the physician interpreting the study.

SUMMARY

Since its conception in 1917, image reconstruction from projections has undergone a number of changes. The simplest technique is basic backprojection, a crude "brute force" attack on image reconstruction, which generates numerous artifacts. Filtered or convoluted backprojection methods are the predominant technique in commercial instrumentation because of their ease of opera-

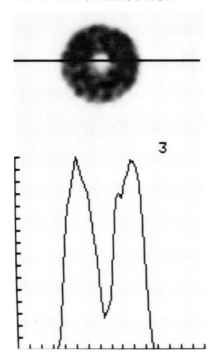

FIG. 2-7. Reconstruction (with no attenuation correction) of a ^{99m}Tc-filled cylindrical phantom and histogram of relative counts. Attenuation of photons seen in the sloped profile across the cold vial in the phantom. Proper attenuation correction would present a perpendicular profile.

tion, implementation, and reduced generation of artifacts. Other more elegant techniques, both analytic and iterative, have been devised, but lengthy computer time has led to limited commercial implementation.

Unlike CT, which is based on the measurement of photon attenuation, SPECT suffers a serious constraint because of this inherent factor. Commercially available attenuation correction techniques such as Sorenson's and Chang's are reasonably effective with large, homogeneous radionuclide distributions but suffer when implemented with multiattenuating cross sections. Iterative techniques designed for specialty SPECT instrumentation are now being investigated with the rotating gamma camera, with the hope that the obstacle of photon attenuation will be removed as a constraint in attempts at quantification.

SUGGESTED READINGS

1. Brooks RA, Di Chiro G. Principles of computer assisted tomography (CAT) in radiographic and radioisotopic imaging. *Phys Med Biol* 1976;5:689–732.

2. Chang LT. A method for attenuation correction in radionuclide computed tomography. *IEEE Trans Nucl Sci* 1978;NS-25:638–43.

3. Faber TL, Lewis MH, Corbett JR, et al. Attenuation correction for SPECT: An evaluation of hybrid approaches. *IEEE Trans Med Img* 1984;MI-3:101–07.

4. Gullberg GT, Malko JA, Eisner RL. Boundary determination methods for attenuation correction in single photon emission computed tomography. In: Esser PD, ed. *Emission Computed Tomography: Current Trends*. New York: The Society of Nuclear Medicine, 1983:33–53.

5. Herman GT. *Image Reconstruction From Projections*. New York: Academic Press, 1980.

6. Kay DB, Keys JW. First order correction for absorption and resolution compensation in radionuclide fourier tomography. *J Nucl Med* 1975;16:540–41.

7. Keyes JW. Computed tomography in nuclear medicine. In: Liberman DE, ed. *Computer Methods: The Fundamentals of Digital Nuclear Medicine*. St. Louis: CV Mosby, 1977:130–38.

8. Moore SC, Brunelle JA, Kirsch CM. Quantitative multi-detector emission computerized tomography using iterative attenuation compensation. *J Nucl Med* 1982;23:706–14.

9. Nahmias C, Kenyon DB, Kouris K, et al. Understanding convolution backprojection. In: *Single Photon Emission Computed Tomography and Other Selected Topics*. New York: The Society of Nuclear Medicine, 1980:19–29.

10. Sorenson JA. Methods for quantitative measurement of radioactivity in vivo by whole-body counting. In: Hine GJ, Sorenson JA, eds. *Instrumentation in Nuclear Medicine*. Vol. 2. New York: Academic Press, 1974:311–48.

11. Tauxe WN, Soussaline F, Todd-Pokropek A, et al. Determination of organ volume by single photon emission tomography. *J Nucl Med* 1982;23:984–87.

12. Todd-Pokropek A. The mathematics and physics of emission computed tomography (ECT). In: Esser PD, ed. *Emission Computed Tomography: Current Trends*. New York: The Society of Nuclear Medicine, 1983:3–31.

13. Zielonka JS. Cardiac tomography. In: Holman BL, Parker JA, eds. *Computer Assisted Cardiac Nuclear Medicine*. Boston: Little, Brown, 1981:445–77.

STUDY QUESTIONS

1. *The backprojected image is*
a. a filtered, processed view.
b. a composite of all the ray sums.
c. a cross-sectional view of the original field.
d. a computer-assisted trans-axial view.
e. b and c.
f. b and d.

2. *A ray sum is best defined as*
a. the imaging path.
b. the overlap projection of a source.
c. density buildup of the counts.
d. an even projection of the source along the path of acquired angle.
e. c and d.
f. none of the above.

3. *The "star" effect can be created by*
a. improper source storage of the points.
b. artifacts produced from the overlapping of the ray sums.
c. septal penetration.
d. patient motion.
e. none of the above.
f. all of the above.

4. *Filtering*
a. cannot remove the "star" effect.

b. introduces a small negative value to the density portion of the ray sum.
c. is basically different for each computer system.
d. will cancel or lose all but the highest density in the image.
e. b and d.
f. c and d.

5. *Data, counts per pixel, can be portrayed*
a. in frequency space.
b. in real space.
c. in a series of sinusoidal curves.
d. in a convoluted reflection image.
e. a and b.
f. a, b, and c.

6. *Fourier transformation*
a. transforms counts per pixel from frequency space into real space.
b. is limited by spatial resolution.
c. equates observed emission values with transverse distribution.
d. is limited by the imaging device's resolution.
e. b and c.
f. all of the above.

7. *Attenuation*
  a. is not a problem with
     SPECT.
  b. as a problem is diminished
     with SPECT, since multi-
     ple views are acquired.
  c. correction methods must
     be used in SPECT because
     the measurement process
     "mixes" the activity
     distribution with the at-
     tenuating material.
  d. compensation methods
     must be applied to the raw
     data before reconstruction
     is performed.
  e. is often demonstrated by
     an area of increased activi-
     ty or only appreciated on a
     high-count study.
  f. c and e.

8. *Accurate quantitative informa-*
tion about radiopharmaceutical
uptake is limited by
  a. patient motion.
  b. dose restrictions.
  c. exponential attenuation of
     photons by the patient's
     body.
  d. a high count rate.
  e. b and c.
  f. c and d.

3 QUALITY CONTROL REQUIREMENTS

Quality control has always been a necessity in nuclear medicine, growing in sophistication as the technology has expanded. From peaking a single photomultiplier tube (PMT) on a rectilinear scanner to loading a uniformity flood into onboard correction circuitry, the integrity of any study has been only as reliable as the quality-control protocol. SPECT brings the quality-control requirements of scintillation camera technology a number of steps further, in both application and necessity. If the reconstructed image in SPECT is to be considered a product of 32–180 separate static projections, any artifacts inherent in these individual static images will be compounded.

INITIAL EVALUATION

The rotating gamma camera installed for SPECT utilization is first and foremost a standard gamma camera and, as such, must meet established acceptance criteria. If one accepts the fact that image reconstruction will magnify standard inherent gamma camera inadequacies, minimum established acceptance standards for a gamma camera must be met and maintained. Upon completion of installation and release of the instrument by the manufacturer, the technologist should evaluate and record optimal planar and SPECT performance parameters as a baseline for future quality-control analysis.

When establishing these base-line parameters, protocols should be developed that can not only be accomplished with existing in-house equipment, and reasonable "specialty equipment" purchases, but be completed within acceptable times as well. Standard planar camera performance characteristics should include measurements of intrinsic spatial resolution, linearity, and uniformity. If records of these easily performed tasks are maintained from the date of installation and routinely thereafter, subtle changes in camera performance can be detected and corrected with a minimum of inconvenience. Planar resolution and linearity may be evaluated by simply calculating the full width at half maximum (FWHM) and full width at tenth maximum (FWTM) measurements of an acceptable line source. The line source may be either a 1-mm-wide series of slits in a lead sheet (National Electrical Manufacturer Association) or a 1-mm-diameter length of pipet or tubing, as long as the techniques employed are consistent. The use of bar phantoms for resolution and linearity testing is not entirely ruled out for these measurements; however, the long-term recording of numerical data as opposed to visual interpretation presents a more reliable demonstration of discrete changes. Evaluation of intrinsic uniformity should be no different than those techniques prescribed by the manufacturer or employed for the nuclear medicine department's other gamma camera systems.

Immediately after installation, evaluation and records should be made of any factor directly influencing the digital planar image, as variances in this image will be compounded in SPECT. Items such as energy linearity, energy correction, x,y image placement of the digital matrix, and collimator integrity should all be in optimal working order at the time of installation and remain so throughout the imaging life of the camera. Routine monitoring of these imaging factors will prevent the technologist from engaging in situations that might, in some cases, be extremely difficult to correct. Examples of such situations are demonstrated throughout this chapter.

While the establishment of optimal planar images at the time of installation is important, the purpose of the rotating gamma camera is for SPECT acquisition and processing. If the user is satisfied with the camera's planar performance, the acquisition

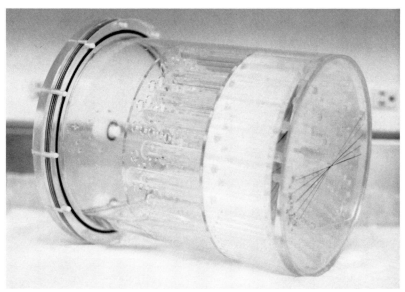

FIG. 3-1. Cylindrical phantom with "hot" and "cold" inserts for evaluation of SPECT performance parameters.

of an "ideal" SPECT situation should be conducted and, if satisfactory, recorded for future comparison. In addition to the purchase of a rotating gamma camera and its peripherals, the user will have to consider the purchase of a cylindrical transmission source for the continued performance measurements of SPECT resolution and uniformity (Fig. 3-1). These refillable cylindrical sources are commercially available and offer the widest evaluation range of an instrument's capabilities. The user's first series of SPECT acquisitions should be dedicated to the optimal cross-sectional display of this source, even if it requires nonclinical conditions. Although acquisition times may be on the order of hours, and the number of acquired projections may be the maximum allowed by the system, the best possible image should be attained as a baseline for future comparison. Upon completion of this exercise, the user should also collect a study representative of a typical clinical situation and should note the significant degradation caused by distance and acquisition statistics (Fig. 3-2). The proper implementation of center of rotation (COR) factors and uniformity correction floods should be performed before this baseline data collection.

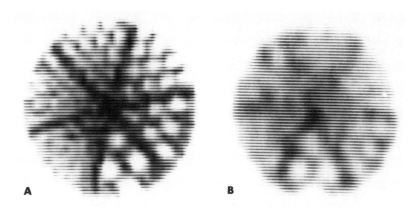

A   **B**

FIG. 3-2. Transaxial slice of phantom, acquired (**A**) with optimal parameters, and (**B**) with clinical parameters.

ROUTINE QUALITY CONTROL

Uniformity Correction

It is apparent from the material presented in Chapter 2 that SPECT imaging is far more complex than conventional planar imaging. While it is imperative to begin with views (projections) of impeccable quality, the added complexities of both multiple data acquisition and sophisticated data manipulation during processing will be magnified during the filtered backprojection process. One of the most prevalent causes of defects in the reconstructed image is gamma camera nonuniformity.

The necessity of a uniform detector field is not difficult to appreciate in standard planar imaging and is easily maintained with state-of-the-art technology of uniformity correction circuitry. However, a variance in field uniformity acceptable to planar imaging may be the source of many artifacts in a reconstructed tomographic image. Uniformity correction is perhaps the single most important quality-control procedure performed in SPECT.

Factors that affect camera uniformity may be either intrinsic or extrinsic, or both. Those factors that originate at the detector include intrinsic nonuniformities of sensitivity and linearity, non-

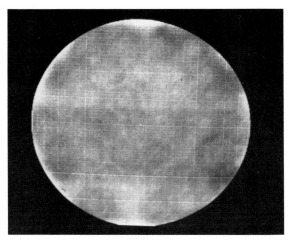

FIG. 3-3. Inadequate differential linearity within the ADC, resulting in horizontal and vertical bunching of counts.

homogeneous response of the camera over the field of view in determining the energy associated with each scintillation event, and variations caused by local magnetic influence on photomultiplier tubes during detector rotation. This last factor, that of magnetic field influence, is not a serious problem with today's PMT-shielding designs. Nonuniformities may also be introduced by differential nonlinearities in the analog-to-digital converter (ADC) and collimator variations.

In some instances, ADCs may be the source of some serious problems (Fig. 3-3). The horizontal and digital lines are the result of inadequate differential linearity or bunching of counts at certain pixels. Analog-to-digital converter problems of this nature can be investigated with the same high-count floods used in uniformity correction. There should be no visible lines in a 30-million-count flood. Gain changes and matrix-offset drifts are additional problems of the ADC. Thus, regular pixel size measurements should be performed, as described later in this chapter.

To appreciate the influence of nonuniformities on the reconstructed image, consider a slight defect on a flood field histogram representative of a detector's field of view (Fig. 3-4). If this reduced area of counts is tracked throughout the 360° radius of rotation, a circular trail of decreased counts will be reconstructed in the cross-sectional image of this flood field, presenting what is commonly called a "bull's-eye" artifact (Fig. 3-4). Furthermore, if we concede that resolution is not the strong point of SPECT and that contrast is, this circular path of reduced counts gains more significance and influence than it had in its original planar view. These nonuniformity artifacts will also have greater influence in the center of the reconstructed image's field of view than at the outer edges, for there are substantially fewer pixels in the center to distribute these defects than there are with each increment radiating toward the edge.

With so many sources of detector nonuniformity as well as improved contrast enhancing even the most insignificant of these regions, the key to reducing the influence of uniformity artifacts with SPECT is to correct the planar projections with correction floods of infinite statistics. The application of this correction process

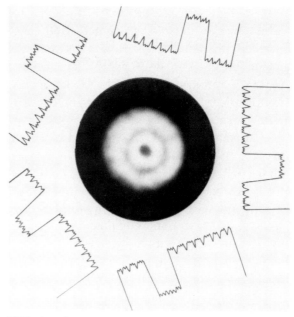

FIG. 3-4. Cross-section of a uniform cylindrical source with resultant "bull's-eye" artifacts that might be caused by the circular path of a nonuniform field, demonstrated by the exaggerated surrounding histogram.

at the end of the projection-imaging chain will take into account all the inherent sources of nonuniformity previously described and reduce the statistical influence of those nonuniform areas that are found in any detector system.

The SPECT software commercially available today enables the user to collect and retrieve a flood-correction matrix of pre-defined total counts. This matrix can be applied either to each projection frame during acquisition of a clinical study or to the complete set of projections at a later time. The flood-correction programs provided by most manufacturers are based on the multi-plicative formula

$$F_i = \frac{\text{mean flood counts}}{C_i} ,$$

where F_i is the correction factor applied to each projection pixel, and C_i is the counts in the ith pixel.

Correction floods of infinite statistics will make the statistical influence of field nonuniformities less significant. Infinite statistics are an unrealistic approach, however, yielding an alternative rule of thumb, "the more the better," with a degree of reasonability being accepted. Standard onboard uniformity-correction circuitry will store and apply a correction flood of 7–12 million counts, which is effective with static imaging. If, however, we consider the prin-ciple that each reconstructed slice will magnify even the slightest defect, the statistical importance of these defects must be mini-mized. Thus, with 10 million counts in a flood image distributed among 3,200 pixels in a circular 64×64 matrix, the average counts are 3,100 counts/pixel. This would generate an expected standard deviation (s.d.) of 2%. A 30-million-count flood would yield an expected s.d. of 1%, one-half that of a 10-million-count flood. Cor-rections performed with a high-count density will yield correspond-ingly lower variations, resulting in a low amplification of artifacts in reconstructed SPECT images.

Figure 3-5 illustrates the inadequacy of an onboard uniformity correction as opposed to a 30-million-count multiplicative correc-tion. A cylinder phantom uniformly filled with ^{99m}Tc, surround-ing an off-center "cold" vial, demonstrates a concentric ring

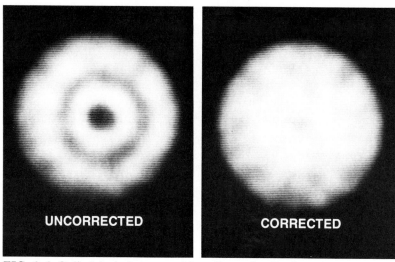

FIG. 3-5. Cylindrical phantom with uniform distribution of radionuclide, uncorrected and corrected with a 30-million-count flood.

radiating from the central axis as well as its disappearance when properly corrected (Fig. 3-6).

A number of issues and questions are raised when considering the acquisition of the high-count flood-correction matrix. A review of several manufacturers' operating manuals reveals a number of radically opposing techniques, predominantly designed to the favorable or unfavorable characteristics of their instrument's energy-correction circuitry. The one common denominator is the high-count flood correction matrix. Most investigators of uniformity-correction techniques agree that the flood-correction matrix should be collected extrinsically to take into account the inherent discrepancies of the collimator. Some manufacturers contend that these extrinsic floods should also take into account the PMT response to those radionuclides that have higher or multiple energy photo-peaks, such as ^{67}Ga and ^{123}I. The user is urged to follow the manu-facturer's guidelines, but for those who prefer not to take any chances, the commercially available refillable transmission source is recommended (Fig. 3-7). The purchase of this type of source allows the user the luxury of predetermining the source activity, energy, and thus the time of acquisition.

If ^{67}Ga or ^{123}I is a commonly used radionuclide in a given laboratory, the purchase of additional refillable sources is recom-

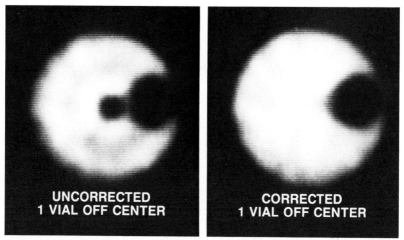

FIG. 3-6. Cold vial placed off-center in cylindrical phantom, illustrating ring artifacts generated from center of the field of view.

mended. This may seem an unwarranted initial expense, but it should be kept in mind that these sources are a one-time-only purchase. One point to consider with these refillable sources is that they can be a source of nonuniformity artifacts if not filled properly. Air bubbles in or bulging of the source may be the cause of some unusual artifacts (Fig. 3-8). A number of techniques have been

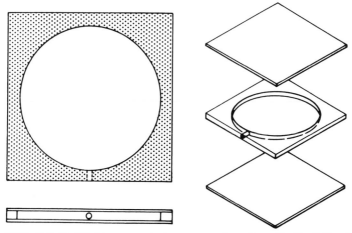

FIG. 3-7. Refillable transmission source that allows for flexibility in acquisition of high statistic flood corrections. (Courtesy of English RJ, Polak JF, Holman BL, *J Nucl Med Technol* 1984;12:7-9.)

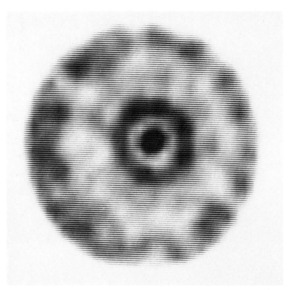

FIG. 3-8. Multiple artifacts generated by air bubbles in refillable transmission source.

developed and reported in the literature. These techniques assure a 1% statistical accuracy in the source, to again reduce the number of factors that might alter the reconstructed image unfavorably. If the length of acquisition time for a 30-million-count flood matrix is of concern to the technologist, the overnight collection of the flood, and the subsequent postcorrection of projection data might be considered.

Center of Rotation

An influential quality-control item unique to SPECT with a rotating gamma camera is one of circular imaging reproducibility. Does the detector observe the same set of parallel lines in the anterior position ($0°$), as seen in the posterior position ($180°$)? Put another way, is the matrix displayed on the left lateral projection the mirror-image matrix of the right lateral projection? It would be unrealistic to assume that an object as massive as a scintillation detector could be rotated around a perfect $360°$ circumference, with the septa of a parallel-hole collimator in exact alignment with its opposing

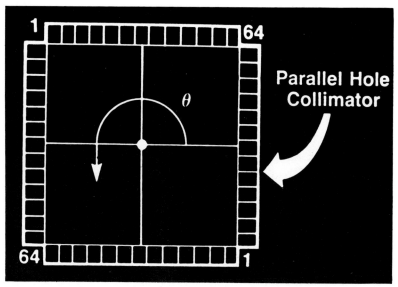

FIG. 3-9. Collimator septa alignment for opposing projections.

view at all angles. Gravity and the mechanics of gears and bearings would prevent this symmetry from occurring consistently. This situation is inherent in any rotating gamma camera system, but its severity and implications can be reduced and kept to a minimum by proper correction procedures.

This problem can be better appreciated if one considers a detector with a parallel-hole collimator positioned in four views at right angles to each other (Fig. 3-9). Ideally, each opposing septa would be in perfect alignment with its opposite number. If the field of view for each of these four views were a 64 × 64 matrix, a point source placed at the exact center would have the ideal coordinates of 32.5, 32.5. If the radius of rotation of the detector was a perfect circle, each planar view would place the point source in this coordinate pair for each of its respective image matrices, and the reconstructed image would be free of error. Since this situation only exists in theory, a correction factor must be used to compensate for any misalignment. The misalignment may be the result of one or any of a combination of factors but can be adequately dealt with if kept within a reasonable range.

The COR provides a method of determining each planar projection's interpretation of the camera's axis of rotation. Variations in this interpretation are corrected with an offset or "error" factor that is effective with the inherent minor discrepancies of the system. In situations of severe misalignment, the offsets provide little or no relief from image degradation. It might also be added that the use of incorrect offsets may contribute to misplacement of counts in pixels throughout the reconstructed image. This situation is illustrated when a cylindrical phantom with "cold" rods is acquired with a correct COR and acquired again with all parameters the same, but with incorrect COR factors (Fig. 3-10). A close look at the reconstructed images demonstrates that "hot" spots are apparent at the "cold" areas. The purpose of this demonstration is to make the technologist aware that COR factors appropriate for one collimator may not be interchangeable in every case because of septal differences.

Center-of-rotation artifacts, or misalignments, may be the result of gradual, long-term degradation caused by the mechanics of the rotating gantry, discrete changes in crystal packing with resulting shifts in crystal placement, or electronic shifts in camera tuning and ADC gain. The importance of recording the initial setup, COR factors, and routine monitoring of these parameters is paramount for demonstrating subtle patterns that might prevent problems of a greater magnitude if left unchecked. An ex-

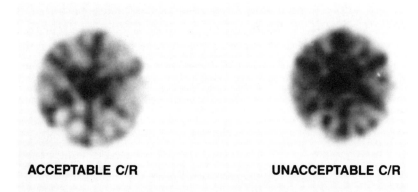

ACCEPTABLE C/R   **UNACCEPTABLE C/R**

FIG. 3-10. Phantom acquired with proper COR factors and improper COR calibration.

ample might be the changes that take place in gantry rotation performance over time. The repeated rotation and interlocking of gears may cause a wearing down or poor contact of gear teeth in isolated locations, inflicting a slight "jerking" effect during rotation. This effect may be mild at first, demonstrating no observable problems in clinical images and only minor variations in COR plots. With time, these minor variations in the COR plot may demonstrate consistency as well as a slight increase in severity. This should send up a warning flag to the technologist. Minor adjustments made by the manufacturer's service personnel can prevent the acquisition of studies that will demonstrate a degradation in resolution over time.

Changes in COR calculations that are immediate may be caused by sudden electronic variances that affect x,y placement of the digital image matrix or may simply represent a user error. For example, inappropriate mounting of a collimator may result in collimator shifts during the detector's circular travel. If a significant change in the COR plot is observed in a single COR acquisition, the technologist should remount the collimator, check for a firm fit, and repeat the procedure. If the errors persist, a call to the vendor's service department might be warranted.

Evaluation of the system's COR should be performed and recorded on a weekly basis for all routinely used collimators. Those collimators not in routine practice should be analyzed for COR discrepancies before being used in an acquisition. Center-of-rotation acquisition and calculation have evolved into a relatively simple operation that is easily completed in 20–30 min per collimator. The manufacturer's operating manual provides a complete step-by-step method for performing this quality-control process. The practice generally consists of simply locating a point or line source within the center region of the rotational field of view, acquiring a minimum even number of angulated projections, and calculating the COR factors of opposing views from the formula

$$\text{COR} = \frac{P_a + P_b}{2},$$

where P_a and P_b are the maximum pixel element in the opposing projections. If this were to be performed manually, the technique

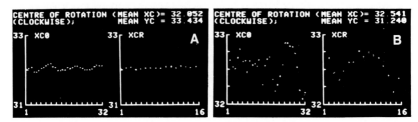

FIG. 3-11. Center of rotation analysis algorithm available through one commercial vendor demonstrating (**A**) an acceptable COR plot, and (**B**) an unacceptable COR plot. The left-hand sides of both **A** and **B** demonstrate the positional deviation of a point/source relative to each projection. The y-axis is the deviation relative to pixel position, and the x-axis is the projection number. The right-hand sides represent the positional deviation relative to opposing projections.

would consist of acquiring a predetermined number of pairs of projections, each 180° from the other, analyzing the point source–pixel relationship, recording the results, and plotting the COR factors versus the acquisition angle. An acceptable detector rotation and one with discrepancies are illustrated in Figure 3-11, with their respective plots.

The above-described technique provides a simple but basic approach to determining the circular travel of the rotating gamma camera. The current generation of SPECT software, provided by the manufacturers, calculates these COR factors, plots the results in a variety of manners, and stores the error corrections for later application during acquisition.

Evaluation of the rotating gamma camera's COR is a unique addition to nuclear medicine quality control and also provides the technologist with a useful tool in the diagnosis of the detector's performance. This procedure should be conducted weekly, a general rule of thumb being that deviations greater than 1/2 pixel will present degradation in the reconstructed image. Most rotating camera systems are able to maintain rotational discrepancies under a 1/4 pixel, with minor variance usually operator induced and major discrepancies a sign of serious mechanical or electronic abnormalities.

SECONDARY QUALITY-CONTROL CONSIDERATIONS

Pixel Sizing

Pixels take on an added depth dimension in SPECT, becoming volume elements, or voxels, but remain subject to the standard planar changes of gain, drift, and resultant degradation of resolution. Monitoring of pixel size should be incorporated in the quality-control protocol on at least a monthly basis. This process can be accomplished by simply determining the number of pixels that represent a known distance. For example, a large field-of-view detector may have an imaging diameter of 43 cm. A 64 × 64 matrix representative of this field would establish a pixel size of 6.7 mm and a 128 × 128 matrix yielding a pixel size of 3.3 mm. To establish that this measurement exists in reality, the technologist simply collects an image of two 1-mm parallel line sources, 10 mm apart, counts the number of pixels between the center of the two line sources, and then calculates the millimeters per pixel. Two line sources, 10 mm apart, represented by a 3-pixel displacement on the displayed 128 × 128 image matrix would represent a 3.3-mm pixel width. Rotating the line sources 90° would provide the pixel width in the opposite direction.

This process should be carried out in all commonly used matrices in the x and y directions and compared with the ideal possibility. The x and y values should be equal as well as stable over time. Changes in these factors would warrant adjustments in the x,y gain, analysis of the ADC, or a call to the manufacturer.

Collimator Integrity

Uniformity, resolution, sensitivity, and overall camera performance are generally marketed as a function of the intrinsic capabilities of the detector; however, the placement of a soft, pliable, honeycomb metal between a source and the detector will degrade all the parameters. The collimator is probably the most taken-for-granted component of a SPECT system; yet it has a major role in the production of quality reconstructed images.

As stated in the discussion of uniformity, the "purist's" uniformity correction techniques should be performed extrinsically in order to correct for those nonuniformities that are inherent to the collimator. These high-count flood images acquired extrinsically may also provide images of discrete collimator defects (Fig. 3-12) that may not be visible with low-count flood images or even through visual inspection. The technologist should be aware that damaged collimator septa will introduce reconstruction artifacts as readily as uncorrected "cool" PMTs, but they will not be as easily corrected. It is recommended that the routine inspection of collimator integrity be conducted both visually and through the high-count extrinsic flood image. If damaged septa are encountered, the user is advised to refrain from further acquisition until the problem is corrected or the collimator replaced.

Image/Matrix Alignment

A number of gamma camera systems allow for the manual placement of the analog image coordinates onto the digital image matrix. Reset buttons are available to provide an automatically centered

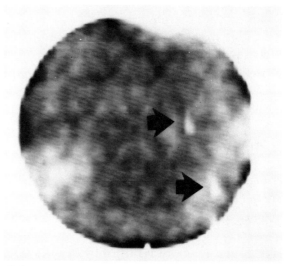

FIG. 3-12. Collimator defects (arrows) and photomultiplyer deficiencies well visualized on 30-million-count flood (extrinsic) image.

matchup, but the routine check of this alignment might save future questionable SPECT performance. In essence, this misalignment may place counts collected at the exact center of the detector field-of-view into pixels 34,36, while the stored uniformity correction floods and COR factors are centered in the 32,32 coordinates. In those cases in which there are radical count changes (i.e., edge packing effects), matrix misalignment will be enhanced in the reconstructed image. Figure 3-13 demonstrates a reconstructed image of a source corrected with a flood correction acquired on an offset matrix. The intense partial edge effect is a result of flood-correction pixels that are count free because of matrix misalignment.

Evaluating the alignment of the acquired-to-displayed image is easily performed with a fine collimated point source. Approximately 5-μCi of ^{99m}Tc is simply placed in a 0.5-ml volume test tube. The test tube is inserted into a lead tube with a 2–3-mm-diameter hole at the bottom. Because this alignment check is performed intrinsically, the lead tube will assure a well-shielded point source. Most manufacturers place a PMT map on the crystal face.

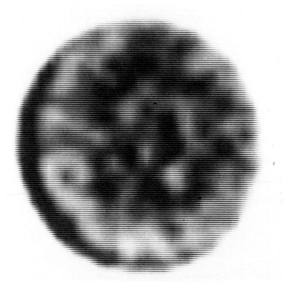

FIG. 3-13. Transaxial image demonstrating edge artifact as a result of unmatched flood correction matrix and study projection matrix.

The collimated point source is gently placed on the center PMT and enough counts are collected to produce an image. The pixel–PMT relationship is analyzed using the computer's profile, histogram, or region-of-interest capabilities. Each software package provides some method of identifying the pixel occupied by a specific count. Once the user is assured that the center of the detector is in the center of the image matrix, any discrepancies should be recorded for future reference.

Table/Detector Alignment

A number of SPECT systems permit the gantry to be moved away from the table for static imaging. When obtaining SPECT images, however, transaxial reconstructions assume that projections are obtained in planes perpendicular to the detector's axis of rotation. It thus becomes necessary for the y direction of the detector to be parallel to the center of the table. This is to ensure that the reconstruction planes are as close as possible to the true planes. The user is assured of this alignment if the distance from the detector to the table is the same in the 90° lateral position as in the 180° lateral position. This simple method of checking the table/detector alignment will also ensure that distance-related resolution will be equal for most projections.

Equally important, when dealing with parallel-hole collimators, is that the detector assembly be perpendicular to the axis of rotation. The result of a nonlevel detector head will be the superimposition of data from several adjoining reconstructed slices. This situation is not easily visualized on the reconstructed image, but it does compromise resolution and may enhance the problems of partial volume effect. Many manufacturers have placed a digital angle readout on the detector assembly, providing a y-direction angle. These electronic devices should be verified, however, with the use of an inexpensive bubble level that can be purchased at any hardware store.

Acquisition Quality Control

Another situation that should be addressed is improper patient alignment or positioning. For example, positioning for a brain scan may result in perfectly positioned anterior and posterior projections, but in the lateral views only part of the brain is in the field of view. The resultant reconstruction would be performed with an incomplete set of data and would be riddled with artifacts. In the acquisition of abdominal or thoracic tomographic scans, every effort should be made to prevent nontarget items remaining in the field of view. This would include the patient's arms, as well as jewelry, belt buckles, and so forth. Unwanted "hot" spots will have a particularly offensive effect on the reconstructed image. When left in the field of rotation, infiltrates of the administered dose will create secondary "star" artifacts that cross the target source. The technologist must be careful when placing the patient's arms out of the field of collection. The reduction of this potential artifact problem may be offset by motion if the patient is not comfortable during acquisition.

SUMMARY

With each upgrade in the sophistication of nuclear medicine instrumentation, increased responsibility in quality control is required. The requirements of quality control in SPECT become mandatory because of the composite nature of the reconstructed image. Minor discrepancies in a planar situation become the cause of major artifacts when composed into a transaxial slice. These problems may be easily avoided by following the manufacturer's guidelines for quality control.

Uniformity variances may be considered the single greatest problem in SPECT, requiring high-count flood correction matrices for adequate statistical correction. In order to obtain this statistical accuracy of the system as a whole, the "purist" must correct for errors of each component. Even if the intrinsic uniformity of the detector is acceptable, a poorly designed collimator might introduce errors. Detectors with poor energy-correction circuitry may require correction of collected data with flood sources of an identical radionuclide. The "no-chance" technique of uniformity correction in SPECT is the weekly extrinsic 30-million-count collection of a properly filled refillable sheet source of the study-matched radionuclide.

The second major contribution of poor resolution and possible artifact generation is inappropriate COR factors. As a result of mechanical, electronic, or operator error, a variance greater than 1/2 pixel will present problems in the reconstructed image. SPECT systems today are generally able to maintain pixel variance under 1/4 pixel, but weekly monitoring of the COR factors for each collimator will prevent poor study acquisition and will possibly predict the onset of a major rotation-induced detector/gantry problem.

SUGGESTED READINGS

1. Croft BY. *Single Photon Emission Computed Tomography.* Chicago: Year Book Medical Publishers, 1986:177–234.

2. Eisner RL. Principles of instrumentation in SPECT. *J Nucl Med Technol* 1985;13:23–31.

3. Greer KL, Coleman RE, Jaszczak RJ. SPECT: A practical guide for users. *J Nucl Med Technol* 1983;11:61–65.

4. Greer K, Jaszczak R, Harris C, et al. Quality control in SPECT. *J Nucl Med Technol* 1985;13:76–85.

5. Harkness BA, Rogers WL, Clinthorne NH, et al. SPECT: Quality control procedures and artifact identification. *J Nucl Med Technol* 1983;11:55–60.

6. Jaszczak RJ, Coleman RE. Selected processing techniques for scintillation camera based SPECT systems. In: *Single Photon Emission Computed Tomography and Other Selected Computer Topics.* New York: The Society of Nuclear Medicine, 1980:45–59.

7. Rogers WL, Clinthorne NH, Harkness BA, et al. Field flood requirements for emission computed tomography with an Anger camera. *J Nucl Med* 1982;23:162–68.

STUDY QUESTIONS

1. *The center of rotation analysis program*
   a. should be performed daily.
   b. interprets the patient's axis of rotation.
   c. compensates for slight misalignments.
   d. should be used with each collimator change.
   e. c and d.
   f. all of the above.

2. *The most prevalent cause of defects in the reconstructed image is*

    a. patient motion.
    b. improper filtering.
    c. incorrect collimator mounting.
    d. gamma camera nonuniformity.
    e. improper parameter setup by the technologist.

3. *Analog-to-digital converter problems*

    a. can cause nonuniformity.
    b. can be caused by inadequate differential linearity.
    c. can be investigated with a high-count flood.
    d. can be caused by the bunching of counts at certain pixels.
    e. will display visible lines in a high-count flood.
    f. all of the above.

4. *The "bull's-eye" artifact*

    a. is a summation of an area of decreased activity.
    b. is built in a circular fashion in the same geometric pattern as the detector rotation.
    c. is most prominent in the reconstruction of diffuse homogeneous studies.
    d. is caused by a variance in field uniformity.
    e. b and d.
    f. all of the above.

5. *A high-count flood*

    a. is recommended for flood correction by all vendors.
    b. can be used to check the proper function of the ADC.
    c. should be collected extrinsically.
    d. requires a large cobalt flood source.
    e. a and b.
    f. a, b, and c.

6. *Center of rotation evaluation*

    a. should be performed monthly.
    b. is needed to check for rotational discrepancies greater than ½ pixel.
    c. will demonstrate the reconstruction field.
    d. should be conducted routinely and with a collimator change.
    e. b and d.
    f. all of the above.

7. *A voxel is*

    a. a vertical picture element.
    b. a pixel with a depth dimension.
    c. a volume element.
    d. a and c.
    e. b and c.
    f. none of the above.

8. *Pixel size monitoring*
  a. should be carried out in all commonly used matrices.
  b. should be performed monthly.
  c. should be calculated in millimeters per pixel.
  d. should include measurements in both *x* and *y* directions.
  e. a and b.
  f. all of the above.

9. *Collimator integrity*
  a. should be checked daily.
  b. should be checked visually.
  c. should only require checking upon delivery of equipment.

  d. should be inspected with a high-count extrinsic flood.
  e. a and d.
  f. b and d.

10. *An evaluation of image/matrix alignment*
  a. is performed with a fine collimated point source.
  b. is performed extrinsically.
  c. is performed to check for the correct placement of counts into pixels.
  d. may confirm the cause of intense partial edge effect or count free flood-correction pixels.
  e. a, b, and c.
  f. a, c, and d.

4 ACQUISITION PARAMETERS

To produce quality emission tomographic images, the fundamental principles required to produce planar images must be employed along with those unique characteristics and principles of SPECT. These include instrument integrity, proper collimation, minimal source-to-detector distance, and sufficient statistics. A number of methods may be applied to these principles, varying among the numerous commercially available SPECT systems. Although each manufacturer proclaims their methods as superior, a quality image remains a product of good basic nuclear medicine technology. This chapter examines those basic principles as they relate to data collection, as well as the possible consequences of inappropriate implementation.

PARAMETER SELECTION

The ultimate goal of any imaging procedure is to achieve optimal resolution within the shortest reasonable period of time. SPECT, however, places a demand on the user to often make alternative selections in the interest of time and count density, although this may go against the concept of achieving the best possible resolution. Both the patient and the technology of SPECT place time constraints on acquisition and make the selection of alternative resolution parameters a necessity. For example, the ideal situation might be one of collecting data from a 10-cm circular organ with no surrounding attenuating media, no table for support, and no time or dose constraints. This situation would allow for the selection of optimal resolution parameters, consisting of a high-resolution collimator, an infinite number of projections in a 360° rotation, and a 128 × 128 storage matrix. Depending on the administered dose, several hours of acquisition time would yield a high-resolution set of transaxial images.

In reality, however, the average patient's tolerance of examination tables restricts the acquisition time to a maximum of 30–45 min, and restricted dose administration will limit any concept of high statistics per reasonable unit of time. The technologist must select those parameters that will best suit the needs of the patient and the requirements of the study, while taking into consideration the standard tradeoff between resolution and sensitivity. An additional consideration not frequently addressed is computer disk space. Before the user selects the collection parameters for a 180-frame 128 × 128 word-mode tomographic study, the amount of contiguous space should be checked. This may save the user, as well as the patient, the distress of waiting for the computer while it tries to squeeze the disk to accomodate this massive storage problem.

MATRIX SELECTION

Achieving a higher resolution by increasing the matrix size is an acceptable practice in standard planar imaging, but it may be the source of some difficult situations and perhaps unnecessary resolution overkill in tomographic studies. In SPECT, a change of the image matrix from 64 × 64 to 128 × 128 results in all aspects of the study being increased by a factor of 4. This four-fold increase would require a substantial increase of contiguous disk space, a cumbersome burden if the disk is in the 12–25-megabyte range. This overall increase also applies to the uniformity correction statistics. If 30 million counts are the statistically accepted minimum requirement for a 64 × 64 matrix flood field, a comparable count density would require at least 120 million counts for a 128

× 128 matrix. Image processing is also affected by this matrix increase, both in time and again in storage space. Reconstructions, filtering, attenuation correction, and reorientation of tomographic data all take longer periods of time, and increased contiguous disk space is again required to store the processed data sets.

The increased resolution seen in a 128 × 128 matrix may not warrant the increased time and space or be needed for a clinical study. The optimal pixel size for a clinical study is usually considered at least one-half the FWHM of the system. In a rotating gamma camera, the FWHM is usually in the range of 12–20mm, requiring a pixel size of 6–10mm. These are the typical limits of a 64 × 64 matrix when representing a large field-of-view scintillation detector. In addition, the counts per pixel will be reduced by a factor of 4 if a 128 × 128 matrix is employed. This will diminish the statistical value of an already photon-deficient procedure.

PROJECTIONS PER ROTATION

Radon's original paper in 1917 stated that a three-dimensional image could be reconstructed from an infinite set of two-dimensional images. The concept of "the more the better"still holds true. In SPECT acquisition, primarily because of the patient's lack of enthusiasm for lengthy examinations, a compromise must be found between time of data collection and ideal statistics, but this compromise does not necessarily have to influence the number of projections. It can be appreciated that the more projections in an arc, the higher the quality of the reconstruction. Figure 4-1 represents a series of three line-source acquisitions and reconstructions. The first collection was acquired for 40 sec per projection with 32 views encompassing a 360° arc. Each of the following acquisitions were performed with a doubling of the planar views and a halving of the collection time. Increasing the number of projections substantially reduced the "star" effect when the reconstruction process was implemented, without any appreciable increase in collection time or reduction in acquired statistics. This method of collection must be used with caution when performing low-count studies, for sufficient counts per pixel should be provided to make the in-

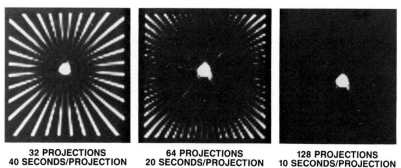

32 PROJECTIONS   **64 PROJECTIONS**   **128 PROJECTIONS**
40 SECONDS/PROJECTION **20 SECONDS/PROJECTION** **10 SECONDS/PROJECTION**

FIG. 4-1. Transaxial slice of line source illustrating reduction of "star" artifact with increase in acquired number of projections.

dividual projections statistically viable. For example, the increased number of projections is viable in a liver study, disk space permitting, but is not highly recommended for the radiolabeled amine brain procedures. It also appears that when collecting data from sources larger than a point, the difference between 64 and 128 projections becomes negligible (Fig. 4-2). From these examples, one may conclude that clinical studies need not use massive amounts of disk space for minimal reconstruction benefits. However, pro-

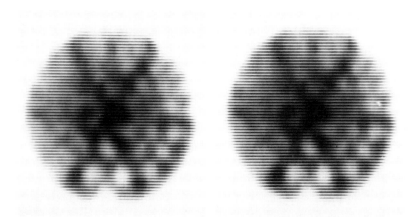

FIG. 4-2. Transaxial slices of cylindrical phantom showing minimal improvement with increased numbers of projections, above a minimum of 64.

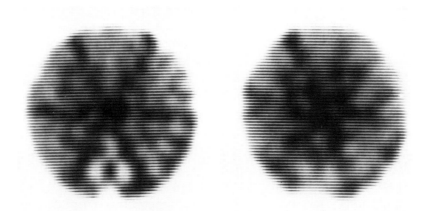

FIG. 4-3. Transaxial slices of cylindrical phantom demonstrating effects of insufficient numbers of projections.

jections numbering less than approximately 60 in a 360° arc may introduce unnecessary artifacts (Fig. 4-3).

ACQUISITION TIMES

Acquisition times in SPECT are subject to the same basic concepts and restraints as standard nuclear medicine imaging. As important a factor as optimal counts per unit area are, the patient's emotional and medical status can prohibit timely completion of a study. The successful completion of an artifact-free quality reconstruction slice is questionable if all ideal collection parameters are implemented—and the patient moves during the last 5 min of the examination.

Most manufacturers provide a recommended formula to determine the ideal acquisition time on the basis of count rate, matrix size, and number of projections per arc. These formulas should be used as effective guidelines; however, the technologist must make the final judgement as to the patient's endurance. This endurance time is then divided by the number of desired views to yield a time per projection. It should be stressed, however, that the key to acquisition times is to make a realistic appraisal of the patient's ability to remain still.

RADIUS OF ROTATION

Throughout this text, the poor resolution of SPECT has frequently been alluded to as a major drawback to a useful technology. The primary cause of this resolution problem is the source-to-detector distance, compounded by body contour. The situation can be appreciated by acknowledging that noncircular objects such as the chest or abdomen do not fit tightly into a circular field. Regardless of how close the lateral projections are to the body, detector distance will increase in the anterior and posterior views. This problem is easily demonstrated with an acquisition exercise involving a high-resolution cylindrical phantom. Collection of two sets of data using the optimal parameters of high statistics, 128 × 128 matrices, and the maximum number of frames permitted in a 360° rotation were performed. The first set of data was collected with a radius of rotation of 11 cm, 1 cm from the circular edge of the phantom (20-cm diameter). The second set of projections was acquired with a 20-cm radius of rotation, to simulate clinical conditions. Both data sets were uniformity corrected, reconstructed with a Ramp-Hanning filter with a 0.5-frequency cuttoff and corrected for attenuation with a Sorenson attenuation correction algorithm. The effects of distance are demonstrated in Figure 4-4.

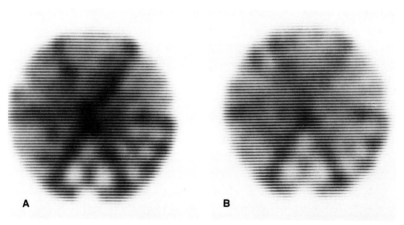

FIG. 4-4. Transaxial reconstructions of cylindrical phantom collected with (**A**) a 11-cm radius of rotation, and (**B**) a 20-cm radius of rotation.

If one acknowledges that the prime cause of the less-than-optimal resolution performance of SPECT is the source-to-detector distance of an ellipsoid in a circular orbit, one could appreciate the benefits of a noncircular detector rotation. Investigations into this concept have been conducted by Gottschalk et al., with phantom studies, demonstrating FWHM improvements of 1.5–2.5 mm and lesion contrast improvements by a factor of 2.8. Two concepts of achieving noncircular data collection are now being investigated by a number of groups: the actual noncircular movement of the detector, and the movement of the imaging table within the circular arc of a rotating detector. Although it is too early to predict the impact of these technologic improvements in the clinical environment, it is safe to predict that improved resolution is a real possibility in SPECT.

CONTINUOUS ROTATION VERSUS STEP AND SHOOT

There are two general modes of detector motion for SPECT with a rotating gamma camera. They are usually referred to as step-and-shoot and continuous rotation modes of data collection.

In step-and-shoot data collection, the camera rotation is under the control of a dedicated piece of hardware—the rotation controller. The controller may be run by the acquisition program, or in some cases, where the camera and computer are from different suppliers, independent of the computer program. The controller moves the camera to successive preset angles. For example, if data are to be taken at 60 angles, a 6° step rotation will be taken by the detector until the 360° of full rotation are completed. At the completion of each step, the computer is commanded to increment until each of the 60 frames of data collecton has been acquired.

In continuous rotation, the detector motion is controlled by a different, simpler controller. It need only launch the detector rotation. The original position of the detector must be sent to the computer program by an encoder that translates the angular position of the detector into a signal read by the data acquisition program. The acquisition is usually set up like a dynamic study with preset time frames and correction for speed variation in detector motion.

When selecting either continuous or step-and-shoot acquisition, resolution and sensitivity should be considered. Continuous motion will cause blurring of the image, since data are being acquired during detector motion. SPECT typically has a resolution of 12–20 mm, and the blurring of a 60-angle 360° study is barely noticeable. On a 120-frame study, it usually cannot be detected at all. Unless very high resolution studies are being performed, the mode of detector motion is not a serious consideration.

COLLIMATOR SELECTION

When collecting SPECT data with routine radiopharmaceuticals, the collimator selection generally follows the same parameters found in planar imaging. The low-energy parallel-hole collimator performs well with ^{99m}Tc and ^{210}Tl, whereas the medium-energy collimator is the best choice for ^{67}Ga acquisition. However, in SPECT studies using ^{99m}Tc and ^{201}Tl the trade-off in sensitivity versus resolution is not as clearly defined as in planar imaging.

Rotating gamma cameras have an inherently poor resolution because of the source-to-dector distance. As a result, FWHM calculations that are tolerated with SPECT imaging would be totally unacceptable in static imaging. By comprehending the distance problem one can easily understand and accept the need to use a collimator with the highest resolution possible. Doing so will bring the resolving capabilities of the system to a somewhat higher level but will still fall short of the average static image. This concept is also complicated by the need for adequate statistics in the limited time available, before inevitable patient discomfort causes movement. The need for preferably high counts in a short time would lead the user initially to consider sacrificing resolution to achieve sensitivity. In two-dimensional imaging, the resolution, collection time, and sensitivity relationship is handled with a variety of accomodating collimator designs. In SPECT, however, a compromise has to be reached to consider all the variables that come with the technology. The low-energy, all-purpose, or general-purpose collimator is the best compromise for this complicated situation when using ^{99m}Tc or ^{201}Tl.

The quality of SPECT imaging is dependent on individual

collimator design for all low- and medium-energy collimators. If the low-energy general-purpose collimator is the choice for ^{99m}Tc and ^{201}Tl imaging, careful consideration should be given not only to hole size and shape (e.g., triangular, square, hexagonal), but to hole length as well. The reconstructed image is a composite of all data collected from multiple projections, including the scatter components. Every effort should be made to reduce this scatter. Those collimators with hole lengths in the range of 20–25 mm may demonstrate excellent sensitivity and adequate resolution but contribute little to contrast. General-purpose collimators with hole lengths in the 40-mm range will improve contrast, retain or improve resolution, and minimally reduce sensitivity. This sensitivity reduction may be misleading, for increased scatter photons yield count rates that are higher and false. The longer hole-length collimators will have sensitivities adequate for SPECT and will also permit the demonstration of a more realistic primary photopeak. This concept is more noticeable when imaging the three peaks of ^{67}Ga with a standard medium-energy collimator. Where scatter from any of the four photopeaks may be the source of septal penetration, the longer hole lengths in a medium-energy collimator will help reduce this problem.

Collimation has so dramatic an influence on SPECT imaging that the concept of evaluating and purchasing them as a separate entity from the SPECT system is well worth considering. A potential buyer should be aware that the finest detector and processing system available is highly dependent on collimator performance, an item that represents a fraction of the system's overall cost.

Collimator selection and performance when imaging with the ^{123}I-radiolabeled amines are critical because of the methods used in the production of the radiopharmaceutical. Iodine-123 is produced from one of two methods: the ^{123}I$(p,5n)^{123}$Xe–^{123}I reaction, or the ^{124}Te$(p,2n)^{123}$I reaction. While the $p,5n$ method yields a relatively pure production of ^{123}I, it is very costly and is not readily available in the United States. It is, however, commonly used throughout Europe. The most common ^{123}I available for labeling amines, a product of the $p,2n$ reaction, poses a considerable number of collimator problems attributable to ^{124}I contamination. Although the contamination is less than 5%, care must be taken when select ing a collimator for brain imaging with the ^{123}I amines. The images can be degraded from the multiple high-energy (greater than 600 keV) photons of the [124]I contaminate. A number of techniques are available to overcome this problem, while attempting to retain sensitivity, resolution, and/or improve contrast.

Low-Energy Parallel-Hole Collimator

Although the 159-keV photopeak of ^{123}I radiolabeled amines lends itself to an immediate choice of a low-energy parallel-hole collimator for SPECT imaging, the [124]I contaminant might warrant a medium-energy collimator. The reduced sensitivity of the medium-energy collimator may be avoided if care is taken to select a low-energy collimator with hole lengths long enough to inhibit the septal penetration of the high-energy photons present in the mixture. This is particularly important when one considers that the greatest concentrations of these photons will be generated from the lung, increasing septal penetration from a source other than the target. Collimators with a septal length on the order of 40 mm will adequately suppress the contaminant's nontarget photons while retaining the much needed sensitivity of a photon-deficient study. In those situations in which only a low-energy collimator with septal lengths in the range of 20–25 mm are available, the better choice for a radiolabeled amine study would be a medium-energy collimator. Nevertheless, the distance problem referred to earlier is present regardless of which of these two collimators is employed. Two techniques are currently available that reduce the distance between the detector and the head and reduce the influence of the [124]I contaminants.

Slant-Hole Collimator

The 30° slant-hole collimator, primarily used in cardiac studies, has demonstrated improved resolution and sensitivity in brain imaging. The technique simply requires rotating the 30° angled septa 180° (cephalad) and tilting the detector assembly 30° cephalad (Fig. 4-5). From a rotational point of view, all collimator septa will be parallel to the source, with the added advantage that the caudate sector of the assembly will be far enough away from the patient's shoulders to have an uninterrupted rotation. Basically, as with the straight-bore collimator, the slant-hole collimator requires that the rotation of the camera assembly define a series of parallel planes perpendicular to the axis of revolution. This whole process permits the center of the detector's field of view to pass very close to the patient's head, producing images that are equivalent to, or better than, those of a straight-bore collimator (Fig. 4-6). This is largely related to the average reduction in distance from 22-cm radius of rotation to 15 cm. Care must be taken, however, to ensure that the collimator septa are true 30° angles. This may be done by monitoring the resolution of a point source, in the y direction, over a 360° rotation. Repeated angulation of the detector until the optimal characteristics of the point source are achieved will provide a true set of perpendicular planes. Many 30° slant-hole collimators are actually within the 26–32-degree range.

Long-Bore Collimator

A prototypical long-bore collimator has been developed that allows for a closer radius of rotation from collimator face to the source. This custom collimator has a 26 × 39 cm field-of-view, with hex-

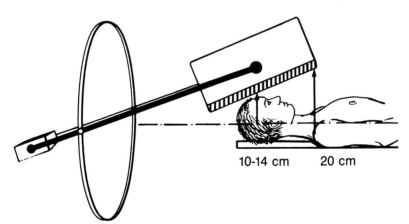

10-14 cm   20 cm

FIG. 4-5. Detector angulation for slant-hole collimator acquisition of a SPECT brain study. (Courtesy of Polak JF, Holman BL, Moretti JL, *J Nucl Med* 1984;25:495-98.)

TRANSAXIAL

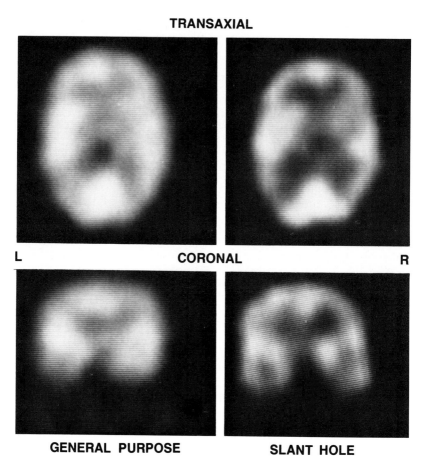

L   CORONAL   R

GENERAL PURPOSE   **SLANT HOLE**

FIG. 4-6. Comparison of general-purpose/slant-hole collimator brain images. (Courtesy of Polak JF, Holman BL, Moretti JL, *J Nucl Med* 1984;25:495-98.)

agonal holes 130 mm long (Fig. 4-7). Although this collimator demonstrates some loss in sensitivity, less resolution loss in the presence of high-energy photons is associated with the contaminant of [123]I. In addition, in collimator design, an increase in resolution is associated with a loss in geometric sensitivity. Thus, the loss of counts experienced with this long-bore collimator can be predominantly attributed to the decrease of unwanted high-energy photons generated from the lungs. This permits improved contrast and, in some cases, improved resolution (Fig. 4-8).

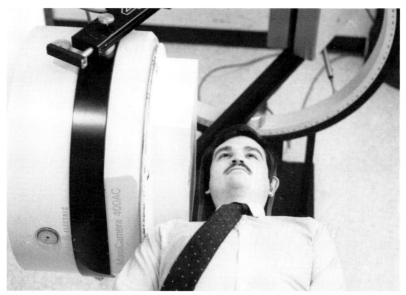

FIG. 4-7. Illustration of long-bore collimator configuration and relationship to patient's head and shoulders.

The long-bore collimator requires some care during patient setup and positioning. The lower and upper portions of the detector face have been eliminated from the useful field of view, increasing the possibility of cutting off the cerebellum during rotational acquisition. Proper centering of the brain on the lateral projection before data collection should avoid this problem. It must also be remembered that both high statistic uniformity correction and COR characteristics must be collected with this or any unique collimator design.

Fan-Beam Collimation

A current collimator design under investigation with SPECT brain imaging is a concept long familiar to nuclear medicine—the fan beam, or custom converging-type collimator. This collimator concept is of two types: the focused-hole collimator with flat detector, and the focused-hole collimator with fan-curved detector. Both concepts use the focusing capabilities inherent in their design to improve system performance. Both system sensitivity and image

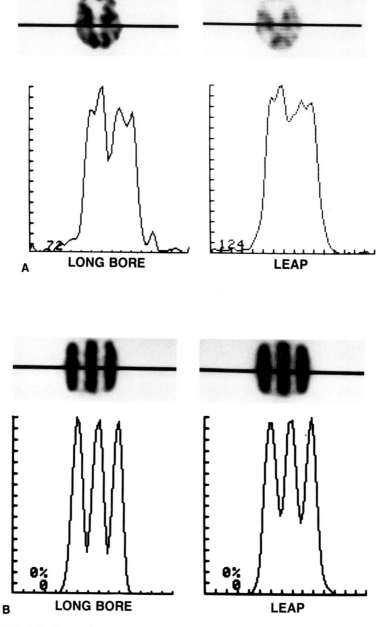

FIG. 4-8. General-purpose/long-bore collimator comparison. (**A**) Clinical brain study. (**B**) Phantom study. (Courtesy of Mueller SP, Polak JF, Kijewski MF, *J Nucl Med* in press.)

resolution can be improved simultaneously with these collimators in combination with large field-of-view detectors. Performance differences between the two types of collimator remain minimal at the moment. Although in their infancy, focus, or fan-beam collimation, holds much promise for improved SPECT performance.

CLINICAL ACQUISITION CONSIDERATIONS

A great deal of material in the literature related to SPECT is based on phantom studies. While these studies are necessary to establish potential problems and promise, they may not always be on the mark in the clinical setting. This section presents a number of acquisition considerations that may be of help when preparing for actual patient data collection. This information is not intended to be ideally suited to every instrument or institution, or both, but merely a point from which to start.

Brain

At first, the brain was the target of choice for SPECT imaging; with the introduction of the radiolabeled amines, the brain is gaining renewed interest. The central problem in brain SPECT, whether with a ^{99m}Tc agent or the ^{123}I-labeled amine compounds, is the substantial distance between the detector and the source, caused by the width of the shoulders. The shoulders can add up to 10 cm to the radius of rotation for a brain study, depending on a given patient's body contour. This problem is compounded with the use of the radiolabeled amines, for two reasons: 1) 25%–30% of the agent is retained in the lungs, generating substantial non-target photons, and 2) production methods of ^{123}I may produce agents with contaminants of high-energy photons (greater than 600 keV) from ^{124}I. A number of detectors and collimator designs have recently been introduced to reduce these problems.

Technetium-99m brain agents adhere to the standard collimation requirements previously described. With the recent introduction of "cutoff/away" detector heads, which allow for a reduced target-to-detector distance, the properties of the straight-bore collimator are retained, while the radius of rotation is decreased. These altered detectors keep the same crystal diameter and thickness, hence field of view, but use thinner detector-shielding properties and designs which result in the reduction of the lower portion of the detector head. The result is a tighter radius of rotation because the shoulders are bypassed. This design provides some advantages but is subject to the length of the patient's neck. A patient with a short neck, or whose head is obliqued to one side will restrict the brain to the outer/lower edge of the useful field of view, thereby cutting off regions of this target in some projections. A different collimator design is perhaps an alternative to the "cutoff/away" head.

Patient positioning is crucial to brain imaging both from a technical point of view and for patient comfort. The use of an extended and elevated head holder (Fig. 4-9) that drops the patient's chin slightly will, in most cases, provide adequate comfort and proper head alignment. Care should be taken to make sure the patient's head is not rotated and is properly positioned in the center of the detector's field of view in the lateral positions, as well as the anterior and posterior views. Patients who are comfortable may fall asleep during this procedure only to be suddenly awakened

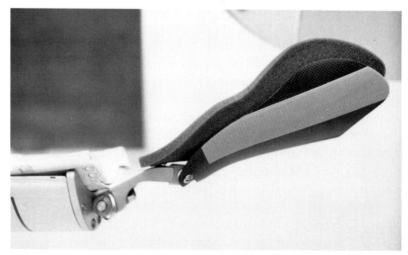

FIG. 4-9. Head-holder design providing positional assistance during brain SPECT.

by some outside noise (e.g., a ringing telephone or conversation), resulting in an abrupt unintentional head movement. The use of a nonallergic mildly adhesive paper tape is recommended for retaining patient position during this long study. This tape will also prove beneficial in preventing the unavoidable subtle rotation of the head and possible lifting of the head into the detector assembly. Both movements are characteristic of those patients who are not fully aware of their surroundings.

Bone

Bone SPECT collection techniques are basically a function of the anatomy being studied. Acquisition of the skull would follow those parameters outlined for ^{99m}Tc brain studies, whereas those parameters sufficient for the liver would be applicable for the lumbar spine. The basic challenge while setting up the acquisition of the chest is the positioning of the arms. If left in the field of view, the arms may produce artifacts; if placed uncomfortably out of the imaging field they may result in patient motion. There is no easy solution; however, the installation of a device at the head of the table that provides the patient with something to hold onto may prove an asset. Such a device does not have to be exotic; it may simply be a cutoff broom handle, or an IV pole, securely fastened to the attached head holder. The region of the pelvis has the inherent problem of a filling bladder. As with planar imaging, the full bladder may overwhelm any surrounding activity, requiring postvoid images. Having the patient void before SPECT acquisition is necessary, but it may not always be the answer. The bladder may fill during the 20–30 min of acquisition time, demonstrating progressive increases in bladder activity from frame #1 to the end. Imaging the lower extremities is uncomplicated when a minimal attenuating medium is placed beneath the knees to ensure that the legs are centered within the rotational arc.

Gallium

Patient positioning for gallium acquisition follows those parameters outlined for bone studies. The most noticeable drawback to gallium

SPECT is the limited number of available counts attributable to restricted dose administration. Currently, a number of institutions advocate an increase in ^{67}Ga-administered doses to provide ample statistics for SPECT acquisition when a triple-peak gamma camera is employed. If this situation is not available to the user, the only solution is uncomfortably long imaging times and their resulting problems.

Thallium

Two schools of thought exist with SPECT acquisition of ^{201}Tl: collection of data with an 180° arc starting from the RAO position and ending in the LPO projections, or 360° acquisition of the complete chest. Those who advocate the 180° methodology point out that the predominant collection of useful data is on the left side of the chest and should be done with as little attenuation interference from the sternum and spine as possible. The 180° acquisition technique allows for the table, and thus the heart, to be raised out of the center field of view, hence closer to the detector, giving the semblance of a noncircular orbit (Fig. 4-10) and increasing statistics while retaining minimal collection times. Proponents of 360° data collection point out that photons originating from the posterior walls of the myocardium are sufficiently ignored during limited rotations to produce potential false-positive studies. They

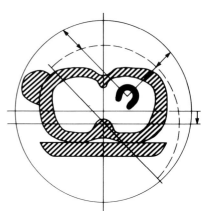

FIG. 4-10. Detector–distance relationship of 360° and 180° myocardial acquisition.

note that reconstruction algorithms are optimal for complete rotations and that the problems of attenuation and distance are not as serious as the incomplete data acquisition experienced posteriorly during 180° rotations.

One aspect of ^{201}Tl imaging, whether planar or SPECT, that is often ignored is the application of the dual peak capabilities of current gamma cameras to collect those gamma photons in the 135-keV range. The addition of these photons will both reduce acquisition times and incorporate a higher-resolution photopeak. Whereas the mercury x-ray peak of ^{201}Tl is the predominant source of counts, the 135-keV gamma peak will demonstrate a noticeable improvement in thallium imaging.

SUMMARY

Establishing carved-in-stone acquisition parameters for SPECT is not a possibility at the present time because of differences in instrumentation, patient populations, and institutional preferences. Appendix B outlines a number of suggestions that may enable the new user to get started, before developing more in-depth custom-designed protocols. Because the technical capabilities of instruments vary, this table should be used with a degree of flexibility and ingenuity.

A number of items pertaining to SPECT data collection can be addressed generically:

1. Source/detector distance must be kept to a minimum.
2. The greater the number of counts, the better the reconstructed image.
3. Patient comfort and reduced motion are a prime necessity.
4. Poor collimation can be the cause of numerous imaging problems.
5. Proper maintenance of contiguous disk space will avoid countless inconveniences.
6. Utilization of dual- and triple-peak capabilities, when warranted, will increase statistics.
7. Acquisition times must be realistic to ensure patient cooperation.

This final item cannot be stressed enough, for the patient is really in control of the study and its successful completion. The technologist must seek to achieve the highest possible resolution, with common-sense collection times, combined with quality patient care and compassion.

SUGGESTED READINGS

1. Coleman RE, Greer K, Drayer BP, et al. Collimation for I-123 imaging with SPECT. In: Esser PD, ed. *Emission Computed Tomography: Current Trends.* New York: The Society of Nuclear Medicine, 1983:135–45.

2. Coleman RE, Jaszczak RJ, Cobb FR. Comparison of 180° and 360° data collection in thallium-201 imaging using single-photon emission computerized tomography (SPECT). *J Nucl Med* 1982;23:655–60.

3. Eisner RL. Principles of instrumentation in SPECT. *J Nucl Med Technol* 1985;13:23–31.

4. Go RT, MacIntyre WJ, Houser TS. Clinical evaluation of 360° and 180° data sampling techniques for transaxial SPECT thallium-201 myocardial perfusion imaging. *J Nucl Med* 1985;26:695–706.

5. Gottschalk SC, Salem D, Lim CB, et al. SPECT resolution and uniformity improvements by noncircular orbit. *J Nucl Med* 1983;24:822–28.

6. Hoffman EJ. 180° compared with 360° sampling in SPECT. *J Nucl Med* 1982;23:745–46.

7. Jaszczak RJ, Greer K, Coleman RE. SPECT system misalignment: Comparison of phantom and patient images. In: Esser PD, ed. *Emission Computed Tomography: Current Trends.* New York: The Society of Nuclear Medicine, 1983:57–70.

8. Polack JF, English RJ, Holman BL. Performance of collimators used for tomographic imaging of I-124 contaminated I-123. *J Nucl Med* 1983;24:1065–69.

9. Polack JF, Holman BL, Moretti JL, et al. I-123 HIPDM brain imaging using a rotating gamma camera equipped with a slant-hole collimator. *J Nucl Med* 1984;25:495–98.

10. Tamaki N, Mukai T, Ishii Y, et al. Comparative study of thallium emission myocardial tomography with 180° and 360° data collection. *J Nucl Med* 1982;23:661–66.

STUDY QUESTIONS

1. *Selection of the acquisition time requires consideration of*
- a. the resolution required.
- b. the patient's ability to remain still.
- c. the speed of the processing software.
- d. the storage capabilities.
- e. a and b.
- f. b and c.

2. *High statistic SPECT studies are difficult to achieve because of*
- a. computer speed.
- b. regulated dose administration and patient cooperation limitations.
- c. collimator design.
- d. patient size.
- e. none of the above.
- f. all of the above.

3. *An increase of matrix size from 64 × 64 byte mode to 128 × 128 word mode for SPECT studies will result in all aspects of the study being increased by a factor of*
- a. 4.
- b. 8.
- c. 16.
- d. 32.
- e. 64.
- f. none of the above.

4. *SPECT typically has a resolution of*
- a. 4–10 mm.
- b. 6–12 mm.
- c. 8–12 mm.
- d. 12–20 mm.
- e. 20–28 mm.

5. *The "star" effect will be reduced by*
- a. less filtering.
- b. increasing the acquisition time of low-count studies.
- c. increasing the number of projections acquired on a high-count study.
- d. increasing the count rate.
- e. none of the above.
- f. all of the above.

6. *The primary source of the resolution problem in SPECT is*
- a. patient motion.
- b. administration of dose restrictions.
- c. the target-to-detector distance.
- d. the poor collimator selection available.
- e. equipment design.
- f. crystal size.

7. *In continuous rotation acquisition,*
- a. the computer commands the detector to increment.
- b. the detector is under command of a simple controller.
- c. blurring is a serious problem.
- d. the original detector position must be sent to the computer.
- e. a and b.
- f. b and d.

8. *Collimator selection should be based on*
- a. the isotope energy and the resolution needed.
- b. the hole length.
- c. the hole size and shape.
- d. a and b.
- e. a and c.
- f. all of the above.

9. *The collimator of choice for I^{123} radiolabeled amine studies would be the*
- a. medium-energy collimator.
- b. low-energy collimator.
- c. low-energy, 40-mm septal length collimator.
- d. medium-energy, 20–25-mm septal length collimator.
- e. high-energy collimator.
- f. convergent collimator.

10. *A slant-hole collimator will be able to demonstrate an average reduction in distance from a _____-cm to a _____-cm radius of rotation.*
- a. 10, 8.
- b. 15, 10.
- c. 22, 15.
- d. 30, 20.
- e. 32, 16.
- f. none of the above.

11. *Iodine-123-labeled amines*
- a. enter the brain matter, where there is a disruption of the normal blood-brain barrier.
- b. reflect local cerebral blood flow.
- c. are retained by the cortex.
- d. cross an intact blood-brain barrier.
- e. b and d.
- f. b, c, and d.

5 PROCESSING TECHNIQUES

The quality of reconstructed images is a direct function of each planar projection. During the reconstruction process, any errors collected in the planar projections are magnified and portrayed in the form of artifacts or reduced resolution. The impact of this artifact generation may be reduced with the application of pre- and postprocessing filters, three-dimensional filters, and, in some cases, alternative display techniques. This chapter deals with the basics of filtering, a few of the options available, the results of correct and incorrect filter applications, and any items generally applied to the postacquisition phase of a SPECT study.

FILTERS

A useful filter is a device that enhances image quality, without significantly altering the raw components of the input data, and that produces results that are easier to process and read. However, overfiltering may produce adverse effects by reducing resolution, accentuating noise, and/or blurring detail in an image. To appreciate the variety of filter options available, one should understand the basic principle of what a filter is and why it is needed in SPECT processing.

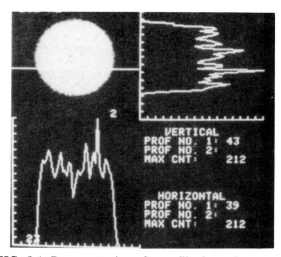

FIG. 5-1. Representation of a profile through a row of pixels. Peaks and valleys represent random-count deviations caused by high-frequency noise and low-frequency background.

NOISE

Noise is a form of distortion that can appear as unwanted contributions to the image from background and/or scatter radiation or as statistical fluctuations in measurements. In planar nuclear medicine, background is most often removed by subtracting average intensities from the picture as a whole. However, the low statistics and composite nature of SPECT require a more comprehensive suppression of background to reduce the "smoothing" effect inherent in filtered backprojection. The method of handling this background noise is discussed further in this section.

Statistical fluctuations in planar imaging are principally caused by the number of gamma photons being measured as a random variable with Poisson distribution. For example, if an average of 400 events are collected in a pixel for 1 min, but in a given minute 420 events are detected, the noise in that pixel is 20 events. This noise can slightly obscure the image signal in planar scintigraphy, but can be the source of serious artifacts in SPECT reconstructions.

FREQUENCY

We are all familiar with spatial domain or, simply put, the counts per pixel or square centimeter. To understand filtering, we must become familiar with frequency-amplitude domain. The conversion from spatial to frequency domain is performed by simply presenting the repetitions of pixels in the mathematical terms of sine and cosine functions. This technique is used exclusively in the form of modulation transfer functions. We might define frequency as the number of peaks per unit distance (pixel to pixel) or cycles per pixel or centimeter.

Consider running a profile through a row of pixels that represent a portion of a 64 × 64 low-count static background image. The resultant plot would reveal a systematic series of peaks and valleys representing random-count deviations across that row of pixels (Fig. 5-1). The sharp, accentuated peaks are indicative of a combination of high-frequency noise and low-frequency background. The maximum number of peaks possible would be in a situation in which noise and background occur every other pixel, presenting a maximum of 32 separate peaks. Thus, the greatest frequency possible for a 64 × 64 matrix is 32, or 32/64 = 0.5. Extending the frequency range beyond this point would only begin

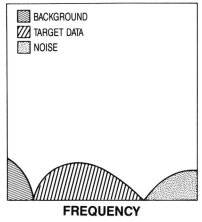

FREQUENCY

FIG. 5-2. An exaggerated, oversimplified example of an image's components in frequency space.

a process of reflection. This point in frequency is called the Nyquist frequency, or that point at which a filter's transfer function begins to fold, that is, becomes a mirror image of itself.

The method of portraying this repetition of peaks is to plot data in frequency domain or to convert the histogram into a curve of amplitude versus frequency (cycle/pixel). An exaggerated representation of the components of an image is illustrated in Figure 5-2. The low-frequency background occupies the far left portion of the plot, with useful or target data in the middle and the high-frequency noise components toward the far right. In reality, data are not so simply distinct as presented in this example, but for our purposes this illustration may provide a better grasp of the filter's ultimate task. The filter selected must exclude background and noise while retaining the useful data.

RAMP FILTER

Filtering software comes in a variety of packages and styles, varying from manufacturer to manufacturer. The one thing common to all their filtering recommendations is the use of the ramp filter in the basic reconstruction process. The ramp filter is that filter (described in Chapter 2) that is used in filtered backprojection. When a point source is projected into each pixel representative of the acquired angle, a ramp filter suppresses the "star" effect. Without this filter, the complete collection of data, including background and high-frequency noise, would be projected as a ray, producing an abundance of artifacts. Background noise, which exists in the low-frequency range, would be included in this projection but would have a smoothing effect in the final reconstruction. With this in mind, the filter design employed in filtered backprojection must not only suppress the radiating spokes of the target but exclude the background noise that will contribute to blurring as well.

One can appreciate that a ramp filter accomplishes this by accepting only data above a specified frequency, thereby excluding the low-frequency components (Fig. 5-3). The ramp filter alone is unusable in routine low-count SPECT studies because it includes

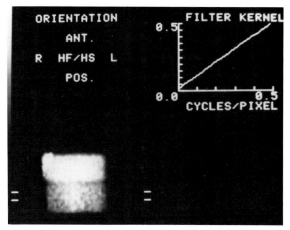

FIG. 5-3. The ramp filter, when related to Figure 5-2, demonstrates the removal of low-frequency background but full acceptance of useful image data and high-frequency noise.

the high-frequency noise component of each projection. If one has a situation in which each projection contains millions of counts, the ramp filter might be acceptable because of the statistical insignificance of the high frequencies. As this is not ordinarily the

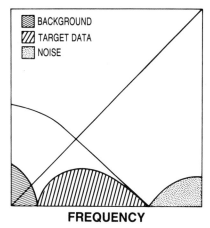

FREQUENCY

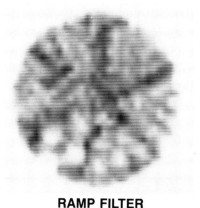

RAMP FILTER

FIG. 5-4. The ramp filter rolled off with a window, to exclude the high-frequency noise, while accepting the image's useful data.

FIG. 5-5. Transaxial slice of a phantom, reconstructed with ramp filter only.

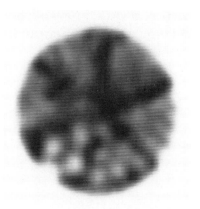

FIG. 5-6. Transaxial slice of a phantom, with ramp filter rolled off with a Hann window.

RAMP/HANN FILTER

case, the ramp filter must be rolled off at some designated point and brought down to exclude the high-frequency noise components (Fig. 5-4). Data that are reconstructed with only a ramp filter are exclusive of the blurring effect of background but are overwhelmed with noise artifacts (Fig. 5-5). If the same ramp-filtered data are rolled off, this high-frequency noise component is suppressed (Fig. 5-6). It must be remembered, however, that the data distribution illustrated in Figure 5-2 does not exist in reality, but is rather an encompassing spread of background, useful data, and noise that is not defined with distinct boundaries. Therefore, a rolloff of the high-frequency noise may easily cut off portions of useful data as well. It is the application of further filtering techniques to this ramp-filtered data that enables the user to achieve the proper balance of noise exclusion and useful data retention.

WINDOWS

Since the solitary use of the ramp filter will greatly enhance the very high frequencies associated with noise, a window function is used to improve the signal-to-noise (S/N) ratio in reconstructions. If, for a moment, we disregard the low-frequency background that is characteristically suppressed by the ramp filter, an ideal filter design might be a rectangular window (Fig. 5-7). This would not only give the best resolution when perfect data are reconstructed but would also accept, and thus amplify, noise of statistical fluctuations.

Since the concept of perfect data is not within the reach of nuclear medicine, this rectangular window may be tailored in a variety of ways to suit the overlap of useful data and the high-frequency noise. A few of these windows are illustrated in Figure 5-8. These window functions share a common ability to alter their frequency cutoff, resulting in suppression of higher-frequency components of data at the user's discretion.

These window functions have a variety of names—Hann, Hamming, Parzen, and many others—but, as can be seen from the plots, they still include the background components of image data. This situation is resolved by multiplying one of the selected windows to the ramp filter for application to reconstructed data. One of the commercially available types of filter-window combinations is the Ramp–Hann illustrated in Figure 5-9. By superimposing this technique on the exaggerated data distribution plot shown

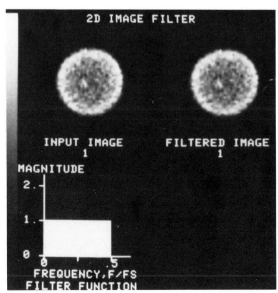

FIG. 5-7. The ideal window, a rectangular window that accepts all image data while excluding noise.

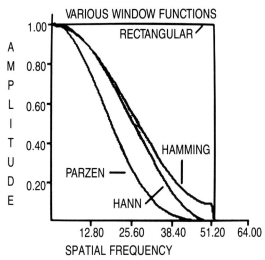

FIG. 5-8. Window variations that may be tailored to include or exclude various frequency components of an image. (Courtesy of Todd-Pokropek A, *Emission Computed Tomography: Current Trends* New York: The Society of Nuclear Medicine, 1983.)

in Figure 5-10, one can easily appreciate the potential advantage of this filter method.

Most commercial software offers the operator a choice of cutoff value selections for this type of filter–window combination. Simply stated, the higher the frequency, the sharper (increased noise component) the image. Reducing the cutoff frequency will increase smoothing and eventually degrade resolution (Fig. 5-11). The best rule of thumb when selecting a cutoff value is: The higher the number of counts in a reconstructed image, the less smoothing (or cutoff) a window function should have.

Many software packages permit the user to apply the ramp–window function during the reconstruction process, primarily to save time and disk space. It is also possible to apply the window function to the raw projections before reconstruction with the ramp filter. When these "smoothed" projections are reconstructed, a simple ramp filter is used during the reconstruction process. If the reconstruction menu allows the user only the option of a

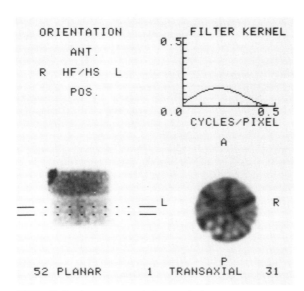

FIG. 5-9. A commercially available Ramp–Hann filter designed to suppress background and noise.

Ramp–Hann, the ramp filter can be used alone by simply entering a frequency cutoff value that is greater than 10. This preprocessing technique is as effective as the combined filter–window application during reconstruction but does require the allocation of additional

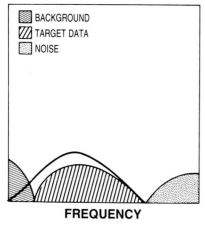

FIG. 5-10. Superimposition of a Ramp–Hann filter over the exaggerated example of Figure 5-2.

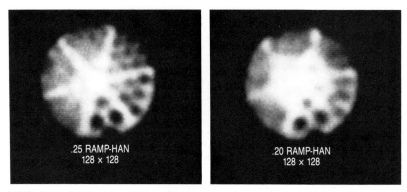

FIG. 5-11. Reduction of cutoff frequency, increasing smoothing, eventually to the point of substantial loss of resolution.

disk space for the refiltered prereconstruction projections.

A variety of filtering techniques are available for varying practical value when all the details of a study's data characteristics are known. For example, the Butterworth filter (Fig. 5-12A) and the Metz filter (Fig. 5-12B) are very design "friendly," that is, easily

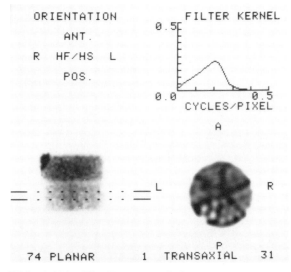

FIG. 5-12A. The Butterworth filter.

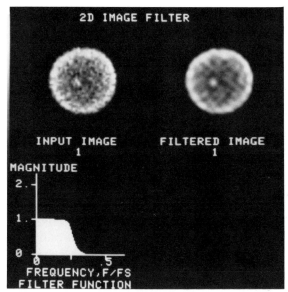

FIG. 5-12B. The Metz filter.

tailored to encompass that portion of data desired by the user. In many cases, these filters will not only reduce artifacts but will also improve sharpness and possibly retain resolution. These filters should be used with a great deal of care and with a thorough understanding of the raw data collected. A reasonable learning exercise is to reconstruct a set of clinical projections using a Ramp–Hann filter with a 0.5 frequency cutoff and then compare these images with those reconstructed with other available windows and cutoffs.

No filter function is perfect—only optimal. The design, acceptance, and implementation of a filter technique will vary from user to user, sometimes at substantial extremes. The best filter is achieved by trial and error, a review of the literature, and, most importantly, proven clinical reliability.

THREE-DIMENSIONAL FILTERING

The original concept of SPECT reconstruction, relating to oblique tomographic display, was a "stacking" of multiple two-dimensional transaxial images to present a three-dimensional impression. The filtering process that worked well for two-dimensional transaxial slices demonstrated streak artifacts in reorientated oblique slices. It thus became evident that preferential smoothing in only two directions (x,y) and subsequent "stacking" of slices would require additional refinement for consistent oblique and sagittal-coronal pixel rearrangement.

To reduce the effects of prominent noise structures (Fig. 5-13), attributable to inherent limited statistics, a number of filtering methods have become commercially available. This software reduces these effects and provides a closer approximation to three-dimensional smoothing. The standard Ramp–Hann, Hamming, or Butterworth filter, performed during the reconstruction process, reduces noise using data in only the x and y directions, while offering no continuity in the z direction after stacking. Alternatively,

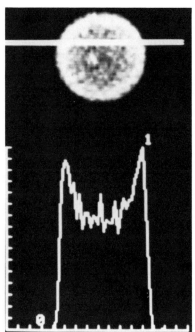

FIG. 5-13. Profile demonstrating noise structure attributable to limited statistics.

planar data may be filtered in the y direction with a spatial filter that has the following coefficients:

$$
\begin{array}{ccc}
0 & 1 & 0 \\
0 & 2 & 0 \\
0 & 1 & 0
\end{array}
$$

after reconstruction of the transaxial data sets, using a Ramp–Hann filter–window with a 0.5 frequency cutoff. This 1:2:1 filter operates pixel by pixel over each planar view, regardless of the slice width and reconstruction limit, and improving the correlation between adjacent slices. With a 64 × 64 resolution, a frequency cutoff of 0.5 is recommended, as the response of the y filter is a close match to the Ramp–Hann cutoff. This technique does have restrictions. This spatial filter is fixed, and three-dimensional planes are rarely invariable.

Another three-dimensional filtering effect is the planar filtering of the raw projections with a 9-point smoothing spatial filter, having the following coefficients:

$$
\begin{array}{ccc}
1 & 2 & 1 \\
2 & 4 & 2 \\
1 & 2 & 1
\end{array}
$$

and then reconstructing the smoothed projection data with a ramp filter. This will provide the same results as the y filtering technique but also suffers the same limitation of a fixed operation.

Ideally, transaxial images should be filtered in all three directions (x,y,z) to obtain maximum reduction in noise structure. Three-dimensional filters are available that apply a smoothing function to pixels in adjoining transaxial planes of the ramp-filtered reconstructions. These filters apply thresholds to reduce noise spikes before smoothing is performed, thereby preserving detail and ensuring slice-to-slice continuity. An alternative method is to apply a two-dimensional variable filter, such as a Butterworth, to the raw planar projections before reconstructing transaxial data with a ramp filter. This method provides a semblance of three-dimensional filtering, while allowing the operator the flexibility afforded by the Butterworth filter.

DATA DISPLAY

Data that have undergone reconstruction are in an orientation that is transverse in relationship to the detector. If the table–detector relationship is in true alignment, the resultant transverse sections through the body will be true for most torso applications. Unfortunately, one of the prime recipients of SPECT interest, the heart, is not in any way related to this transverse plane, presenting reconstructions that are of little diagnostic value. This situation is rectified by a rearrangement of pixels that will present the reconstructed data in any number of oblique orientations.

The new user will find that the implementation of oblique, sagittal, or coronal algorithms takes very little time as compared with initial reconstruction of the transaxial data, as the reorientation software simply rearranges the display format of existing processed data. Data in each pixel element have already undergone filtering, attenuation correction, and other necessary steps during the reconstruction process. This rearrangement may be better understood if one considers the set of transaxial images as a cube, with the x and y planes representing the cross-sectional 64×64 matrix of each slice, and the z direction indicative of the total number of slices in the transaxial file (Fig. 5-14). The maximum number of transaxial slices that can be compiled in this z direction, if the transaxial slices are of a 1-pixel-slice thickness, is 64. If the detector is circular, the number of useful pixels in the upper and lower portions of the cube will be reduced.

If one imagines suspending a heart in this cube, in a position

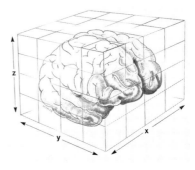

FIG. 5-14. Illustration of a brain positioned in a cube, representative of the x,y,z configuration of stacked transaxial slices.

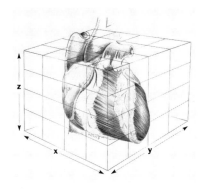

FIG. 5-15. Illustration of the heart in a cube indicative of parallel and perpendicular planes of the thorax, and the necessity of oblique reconstructions.

that may be equivalent to that of a typical study, it is easy to appreciate that the transaxial plane has little to offer in terms of anatomic reference. If those pixels that make up an oblique-angled plane were identified and regrouped, a series of slices could be obtained that represent the long axis of the heart, or that region from the base to apex (Fig. 5-15).

Somewhat less technically imposing is the formation of sagittal and coronal slices. If the brain, for example, is positioned correctly during acquisition, its resultant placement in the cube will require simply peeling back layers of the x,y matrix (sagittal). Sagittal/coronal sections are not just restricted to the brain, but often prove useful in imaging anatomy located elsewhere (Chapter 6).

Oblique reorientation need not be limited to the heart. Oblique protocols may be very effective in obtaining true transaxial views from brain studies that were not collected under ideal positioning conditions. One commercially available thallium protocol is very effective in straightening the rotated brain (Fig. 5-16A), obtaining a more perpendicular vertex position from an extended head (Fig. 5-16B), and forming a well-positioned set of transaxial images (Fig. 5-16C). These techniques may be used to reconstruct any target that is not perpendicular or parallel to the detector plane, such as the acetabulum, temporal regions of the brain, or the patient's congenital variances.

Two considerations must be accepted with display reorientation. A rearrangement of pixels will produce a smoothing effect

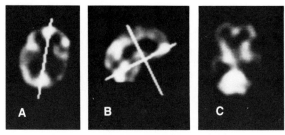

FIG. 5-16. (**A**) Rotated transaxial slice, with positional plane marked for perpendicular reorientation. (**B**) Sagittal view with positional plane identified for horizontal, and thus true transaxial, reorientation. (**C**) Final transaxial view after corrections for poor patient position during acquisition.

and minor loss of resolution and, in the case of thallium exercise/redistribution studies, user-selected planes must be consistent. Figure 5-17 illustrates the operator's ability to place a perfusion defect incorrectly within the walls of the myocardium, with inconsistent processing methodology.

Limiting the effects of smoothing may be achieved through the use of alternative filtering methods on the original transaxial reconstructions. Increasing the frequency cutoff of the window

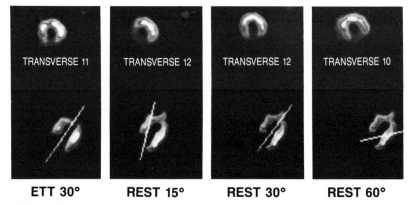

FIG. 5-17. Results of inconsistent reorientation methodology during exercise/rest thallium processing. The region of decreased distribution may be inaccurately placed within the walls of the left ventricle.

function or using three-dimensional filtering techniques on a ramp-filtered transaxial slice may prove beneficial in reorientation display techniques.

QUANTITATION

The quantitative measurement of radioactivity concentrations is one of the major goals of SPECT. In terms of quantitation, we need to differentiate relative and absolute quantitation. Absolute quantitation measures the radioactive concentration in millicuries (Becquerels) per volume element. As yet, this has only been accomplished in phantom studies and is currently subject to extensive research for the in vivo application. Relative quantitation is more easily accomplished, since the configuration of the attenuating medium (i.e., the body around the source) stays the same for all the measurements that are compared with each other.

This is shown in the formula

$$\text{Ratio} \quad = \quad \frac{\text{Image 1 } (x,y) \bullet \text{Atten } (x,y)}{\text{Image 2 } (x,y) \bullet \text{Atten } (x,y)} \ .$$

Calculating a ratio means that the attenuation term cancels out in the equation. Relative quantitation of the change in radionuclide uptake over time can readily be performed.

Much of the diagnostic information in nuclear medicine can be derived from the time course of radionuclide uptake. Using SPECT imaging, the superimposition of structures, and thus the individual organ, can be resolved. This improves uptake measurements. Currently in SPECT, there are two major applications of relative quantitation: [201]Tl exercise/redistribution imaging, and the ^{133}Xe assessment of regional cerebral blood flow.

The most popular technique of assessing myocardial blood flow with quantitation is ^{201}Tl SPECT. By comparing the study immediately after exercise with the one done 3 or 4 hr later, one can visually and digitally diagnose transient ischemia or scar tissue. For more advanced applications, however, such as therapy control after bypass surgery, or PTCA, the relative quantitation to describe myocardial ^{201}Tl kinetics is desirable.

The methods currently employed are all derived from techniques already widely used in the evaluation of planar studies. An elegant solution to the problem of relative quantitative assessment of thallium studies was recently introduced by Garcia, using the bull's-eye display. This sort of display depicts the whole myocardial area in one image without superimposing other structures. Applied to the exercise and redistribution, study parameters such as washout and redistribution can be calculated.

A prerequisite for this type of measurement is that the tomographic studies be comparable. Care must be taken to position the patient for the redistribution study as closely as possible to the exercise study. The reconstruction process employs sophisticated mathematics that place a considerable burden on the nuclear medicine computer system in terms of computing power, and therefore time. Many manufacturers have taken shortcuts to speed up the reconstruction process by scaling the data. If two tomographic studies are to be evaluated by relative quantitation, care must be taken to ensure that both studies either use the same scaling factor or that a cross-normalization can be performed so that both studies will be comparable. In addition, a similar spatial resolution in the tomographic plane, as well as between planes, is desirable. This is achievable with volume-smoothing techniques.

Figure 5-18A demonstrates an example of quantitative ^{201}Tl

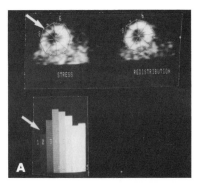 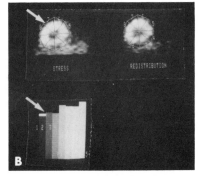

FIG. 5-18. Thallium SPECT images ("cucumber slice") at exercise and rest of patients who underwent PTCA treatment. Images demonstrating decreased perfusion and decreased quantitative index (arrows), (**A**) pretreatment, (**B**) post-PTCA therapy.

SPECT for therapy control after PTCA. The left side shows the evaluation of sagittal slices before PTCA, noting the decreased redistribution in sectors 6–8 of the anterior wall. On the right (Fig. 5-18B), the same patient, evaluated after PTCA, shows considerable improvement.

Another application of quantitative SPECT currently receiving a great deal of interest is the noninvasive measurement of regional cerebral blood flow (rCBF) with inhalation of ^{133}Xe. Although not practical at the moment with a single-detector rotating gamma camera, promising results have been reported with an instrument with four rotating detector banks that acquire three noncontiguous slices at a time. The fast rotation (6 rpm) and the high sensitivity (17,000 cps-μCi-1-ml-1) measured with ^{99m}Tc permit rapid recording of tomographic slices. Because of the speed and the capability of following rapid changes in activity, this method is also referred to as dynamic SPECT (dSPECT).

A study of rCBF takes 4 min: 1 min of ^{133}Xe inhalation and 3 min of exhalation. During each minute, three tomographic slices

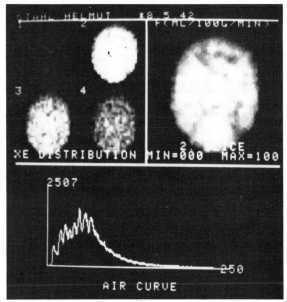

FIG. 5-19. Flow map of cerebral blood flow with SPECT and ^{133}Xe.

are acquired and, with the help of the lung curve recorded by a probe, the final flow map for each slice is computed. As in ^{201}Tl quantitative SPECT, the time course of the radioactivity in all the slices is evaluated in a relative quantitative fashion. Figure 5-19 illustrates a compilation of the input as well as the final flow map for the second of the three slices. On the left, the four tomographic slices of minutes 1–4 are depicted with the air curve over the lung below. On the right-hand side, the final flow map is displayed with its calibration in milliliters per 100 grams per minute of cerebral blood flow.

The relative quantification of ^{201}Tl studies is but one step in quantitative evaluation of SPECT studies. New agents may provide additional diagnostic information if the uptake over time can be included in the diagnostic assessment as seen with ^{133}Xe dSPECT.

SUMMARY

A great deal of attention is given to quality control and acquisition techniques when discussing SPECT. While these factors are crucial to SPECT imaging, they account for only a portion of the complete SPECT procedure. Proper application of filters, windows, attenuation correction, and image orientation converts the raw data from a set of noisy planar projections into cross-sectional images. This technique is totally different from any other previously used in nuclear medicine.

The most common reconstruction techniques employ a ramp filter, which is effective in reducing low-frequency background statistics but which amplifies the high-frequency noise. Because clinical nuclear medicine procedures are count-deficient, the statistical impact of this high-frequency noise will overwhelm the reconstructed image. For this reason, the ramp filter must be modified, or rolled off, with a window, thereby excluding as much high-frequency noise as possible. A number of operator-dependent window functions are commercially available, with the Hann being the most popular.

In a number of instances, the target of interest is anatomically misaligned with the perpendicular and parallel planes of the transaxial planes, requiring reorientation of the stacked transaxial data. These oblique reconstruction techniques will produce some resolution degradation and excess smoothing, requiring alternative three-dimensional filtering techniques. In addition, reorientation procedures must use consistent methodology during repeat studies, such as exercise/redistribution cardiac studies.

Whereas SPECT brings the goal of quantitation in nuclear medicine one step further, absolute quantitation remains effective primarily in phantom studies. Relative quantitation is an accepted technique in a few SPECT procedures, most noticeably in ^{201}Tl studies. Further investigations with attenuation correction and acquisition technology may improve the prospects for both absolute and relative quantitation.

SUGGESTED READINGS

1. Buell UE, Moser A, Kirsch CM, et al. 133-Xe-DSPECT (dynamic single photon emissions CT). *Fortschr Rontgenstr* 1983;139:351-58.

2. Gullberg GT, Budinger TF. The use of filtering methods to compensate for constant attenuation in single photon emission computed tomography. *Biomed Eng* 1981;28:142-57.

3. Han KS, Song HB. Oblique angle display. In: Esser PD, ed. *Emission Computed Tomography: Current Trends.* New York: The Society of Nuclear Medicine, 1983:177-91.

4. King MA, Schwinger RB, Doherty PW, et al. Two-dimensional filtering of SPECT images using the Metz and Wiener filters. *J Nucl Med* 1984;25:1234-40.

5. Kirsch CM, Doliwa R, Buell UE, et al. Detection of severe coronary heart disease with Tl-201: Comparison of resting single photon emission tomography with invasive arteriography. *J Nucl Med* 1983;-24:761-67.

6. Nahmias G, Kenyon DB, Kouris K, et al. Understanding convolution back projection. In: *Single Photon Emission Computed Tomography and Other Selected Computer Topics.* New York: The Society of Nuclear Medicine 1980:19-29.

7. Todd-Pokropek A. The mathematics and physics of emission computed tomography (ECT). In: Esser PD, ed. *Emission Computed Tomography: Current Trends.* New York: The Society of Nuclear Medicine 1983:3-31.

STUDY QUESTIONS

1. *Filtering*
   a. alters the raw data to enhance image quality for interpretation.
   b. by temporal software techniques is the only way to smooth the edges of a low-count study.
   c. manipulates processed images from storage for ease of viewing.
   d. can only be performed with hardware algorithms.
   e. a and c.
   f. b and c.

2. *"Overfiltering" can cause a*
   a. smoothing out of useful data.
   b. superimposition of useful data.
   c. loss of resolution.
   d. frequency cutoff loop.
   e. a and c.
   f. a, b, and c.

3. *The filter algorithm selected depends on*
   a. the interpreting physician's preference.
   b. the target-to-nontarget ratio.
   c. the statistic level per planar view.
   d. the background/noise level.
   e. a, b, and d.
   f. all of the above.

4. *A ramp filter eliminates*
   a. background noise.
   b. high-frequency counts.
   c. low-frequency counts.
   d. a and c.
   e. b and c.
   f. all of the above.

5. *The higher the number of counts in a reconstructed image,*
   a. the more filtering will be needed.
   b. the less smoothing the window function will need.
   c. the more smoothing the window function will need.
   d. then fewer filters will be needed.
   e. a and c.
   f. none of the above.

6. *When selecting the cutoff value for a filter/window,*
   a. the lower frequency cutoff gives less smoothing to the image.
   b. the lower the frequency cutoff, the sharper the image.
   c. the higher the frequency cutoff, the sharper the image.
   d. the higher the frequency cutoff, the more noise in the image.
   e. a and b.
   f. c and d.

7. *If the reconstruction computer menu offers the option of a Ramp-Hann filter, but if you wish to use the ramp filter alone, you would enter*

a. no frequency cutoff value.

b. 0.5 frequency cutoff value.

c. 0.1 frequency cutoff value.

d. 1.0 frequency cutoff value.

e. a frequency value greater than 1.

f. none of the above.

6 CLINICAL APPLICATIONS

SPECT is undergoing a major acceleration in clinical investigation. Beginning with Kuhl's first description of analog backprojection techniques, the brain has been the prime recipient of SPECT interest. Now, with the introduction of radiolabeled amines, a revival of investigative efforts has occurred with this organ. The key to the future success and general acceptance of SPECT may be its demonstrated value in complementing routine nuclear medicine procedures.

A number of clinical studies lend themselves to the unique cababilities of SPECT. The significance of removing over- and underlying structures in gallium imaging is easily appreciated and is only just beginning to be seriously investigated. This concept is also gaining interest in bone scintigraphy and is adding new possibilities to liver studies. The most favorably accepted use of SPECT by the nuclear medicine and radiology community to date appears to be in myocardial perfusion imaging of ^{201}Tl. While researchers pursue the possibility and potential of absolute and/or relative quantitation of myocardial disease, standard visualization of cross-sectional slices of the left ventricle makes believers out of the most adamant skeptics.

This chapter reviews only a few of the current applications and investigations of the possibilities of SPECT, acknowledging that what is in the literature to date is only the tip of the iceburg.

An introduction to cross-sectional anatomy is also provided in order to orient the new user to a different perspective of nuclear medicine anatomy.

CROSS-SECTIONAL ANATOMY

The nuclear medicine technologist has been well trained in the anatomy of planar images. The technologist can identify organs and structures, knows whether they are appropriately centered and whether the projection is correct, and knows how to use surface landmarks in positioning the patient for the appropriate view.

SPECT requires new rules for orientation, since images are now created in a narrow plane at right angles to the camera and reconstructed in variously directed slices that may or may not be at right angles (orthogonal) to the initial plane. It is easier to think of each tomographic image as representative information from a slice of predetermined width through a patient.

Tomographic images have the advantage of presenting structures in an optimum relationship to one another and increasing contrast between target and nontarget areas. There is a price for this, however. The identifying landmarks usually seen in a third dimension are gone, the spatial resolution is degraded, and the image is more susceptible to artifacts that may be misinterpreted as normal or abnormal structures. The technologist must acquire an understanding of how normal structures appear and disappear as image planes through the body are displayed.

Nomenclature of Planes

As defined in Taber's *Cyclopedic Medical Dictionary*, a plane is a flat surface formed by making a cut, imagined or real, through the body or part of it. Planes are used as points of reference by which positions of parts of the body are indicated. In the human subject, all planes are based on the body being in an upright anatomic position.

Standard nomenclature and orientation for tomographic images are important for accurate and efficient interpretation.

SPECT images are usually acquired by rotating the imaging device in a circle, ellipse, or arc centered on the long axis of the body. The initial tomograms are therefore in a transverse plane (Fig. 6-1), which is perpendicular to that axis. Physicians are often comfortable with these sections, since they are similar to those primarily used for x-ray and nuclear magnetic resonance (NMR) imaging.

Two planes parallel to the long axis are also commonly used. One is a section through the body from front to back, which is called the sagittal plane if it is in the midline or the parasagittal plane when it is to the right or left. The other is a section from side to side, referred to as the frontal or coronal plane (Fig. 6-2).

Conventions for displaying these cross sections were first developed during the 1970s with the emergence of ultrasound and CT imaging. While the initial effort was to establish universal standards for all cross-sectional images, it was found that the various specialty groups could not concur on the ideal display orientation format. Presumably, most SPECT images will adhere to the standard conventions as far as possible.

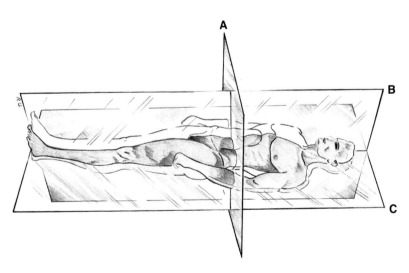

FIG. 6-1. Tomographic planes of the body. (**A**) Transverse. (**B**) Sagittal. (**C**) Coronal.

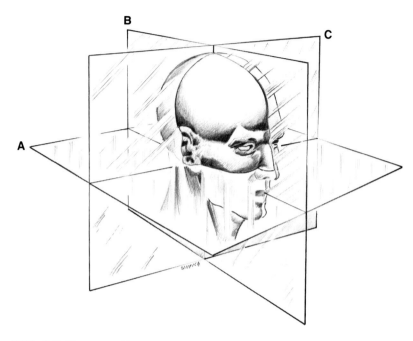

FIG. 6-2. Tomographic planes of the head. (**A**) Transverse. (**B**) Sagittal. (**C**) Coronal.

Standard Orientations

The conventional transverse cross section is presented with the anterior surface up and the right side on the left (Fig. 6-3). It is as though one were facing a recumbent patient from the patient's right side, looking up from below. This is the position most commonly employed by a physician at the bedside. The major exception is in the brain, for which neurosurgeons, who usually operate from above, insist that the left side be presented on the left side of the scan. When a series of transverse sections is presented, they should be shown from above down.

Coronal sections are conventionally presented with the upper portion on top and the right side on the left, as though one were facing a standing patient. This contravenes the long-standing practice in nuclear medicine of looking at the posterior sections as though one were in back (i.e., the left side on the left), but it does match the anterior views. A sequence of sections should be presented from front to back.

Sagittal or parasagittal sections are usually visualized from the right, either upright or recumbent. If upright, the top will be up and the anterior surface on the right. If recumbent, the top is on the left, and the anterior surface is up. Echocardiographers, who examine the heart from the left, have preferred a convention in which the top is on the right, but it is not clear that this orientation will carry through to other modes of cross-sectional cardiac imaging. A series of sagittal images should go from right to left.

The three-dimensional nature of SPECT reconstruction when a gamma camera is employed permits the creation of a large array of oblique planes. Such planes are most useful when the axis of an organ is not perpendicular to any of the orthagonal planes described above. For example, the long axis of the heart runs from the crux to the apex, going inferiorly, anteriorly, and to the left. Cross sections that cut transversely through an organ, although obliquely through the body, are often colloquially called cucumber

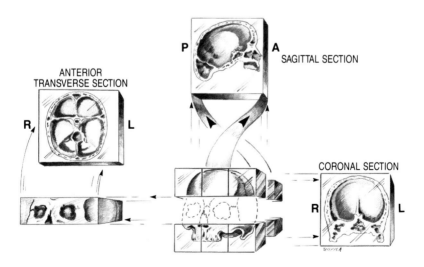

FIG. 6-3. Conventional orientation of cross sections.

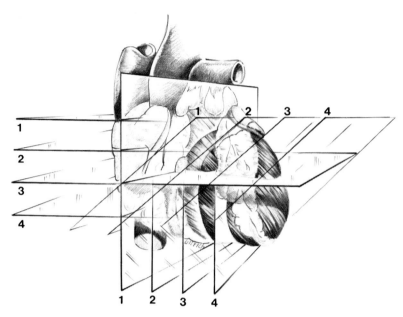

FIG. 6-4. Oblique cucumber-slice cross sections of the heart.

slices (Fig. 6-4). Unfortunately, no universal conventions for naming or displaying oblique sections have yet been developed. For the moment, it is probably best to use the conventions of the orthogonal plane, which the oblique slice most closely resembles.

Anatomic Examples

Technologists wishing to develop their skills in identifying cross-sectional images have received some help from the fact that planar images have some tomographic characteristics because of the following: (a) decrease in resolution with distance because of the collimator; and (b) the decrease in sensitivity because of attenuation. A lateral planar view of the lung looks a great deal like a parasagittal view. An anterior planar image of the liver resembles an anterior coronal section. A vertex view of the skull looks like a high transverse section. A cranially tilted left anterior oblique thallium myocardial image is similar to an oblique cucumber slice.

Clues to the location of a section can come from right-angle images in which the level has been appropriately marked, from regularly spaced sequential sections in which the distance between slices is known, and from common anatomic landmarks unique to each type of scan and plane. The first two aids are simply a matter of good imaging practice; the last requires some experience, which will be illustrated with examples.

Bone Scan. Ribs and vertebral bodies are difficult to pinpoint precisely on transverse bone scans of the torso; therefore, other structures must be used. A section showing the top of the acromion of the scapulae posteriolaterally, and the lateral portion of the clavicles anteriolaterally, is usually at about the level of the seventh cervical vertebra. The glenoid fossa and the head of the humerus appear at about the first thoracic (T1) level. The clavicles approach the midline at T2, join the sternum at T2–3, and are no longer visible at T4. At about T4–5, the wide manubrium transforms into the narrow body of the sternum. At T5–6, the thick knob at the anterolateral border of the scapula disappears, and T7 is usually the lowest extent of the inferior angle of the scapula. The xiphoid process of the sternum ends at about T10.

The lowest thoracic and upper lumbar levels can often be identified by their relationship to the kidneys. Because of variability in their location, these levels should first be worked out on planar or coronal views. Typically, the kidneys extend from about T11 to L3, with the center of their sections moving more laterally and anteriorly from above down. The left kidney is more often higher than the right. Anterior ribs are usually absent below T12 and posterior ribs below L2.

Identification of levels becomes much easier when the top of the iliac crests is reached at about L4. L5 is characterized by well-developed iliac wings, but there is no connection between the ilium and the spine. The appearance of the sacroiliac joints identifies the sacrum. The relatively anterior sacroiliac joint at S1 has moved posteriorly at S3. S4 and S5 appear with the tops of the acetabulae and femoral heads. The coccyx, pubic rami, and femoral necks appear at approximately the same level. The ischia then appear as separate structures medially and slightly posterior to proximal femurs. In the lowest pelvic sections, the inferior ischial rami are seen sweeping anteromedially to the lowest portion of the pubic symphysis.

Brain Scan. Another anatomic example can be taken from brain scanning. The standard CT sections are transverse cuts with about a 30° caudal tilt. We will, however, consider the coronal sections. The most anterior views are characterized by the relatively small volume of the frontal lobes. Approximately one-fourth of the distance posteriorly, the anterior horns of the lateral ventricles appear near the center of the image. Moving slightly farther back, the front of the temporal lobes appears inferolateral to the frontal lobes. Still slightly more posterior, but anterior to the midpoint, the third ventricle may be identified in the midline, inferior to the lateral ventricles.

The midplane roughly corresponds to the (invisible) Sylvian fissure, which separates the frontal and parietal lobes. In this section, the anterior tips of the temporal horns of the lateral ventricles may appear inferolaterally in the middle of the temporal lobes. Just behind the midplane, the brain stem is seen extending downward in the midline. Approximately two-thirds of the distance to the back, the rounded structures of the cerebellum replace the elongated brain stem at the inferior border. At this level, the prominent bodies of the lateral ventricles are only a short distance above the tentorium, which separates the cerebellum from the cerebral hemispheres. The occipital horns of the lateral ventricles characterize the posterior sections, ending only a short distance before the final tomograms through the occipital lobes.

Liver/Spleen Scan. A third example will consider transverse sections through the abdomen on a reticuloendothelial scan of the liver and spleen (see Fig. 6-5). The relative height of the liver and spleen is quite variable and is therefore considered separately. The first appearance of the liver is usually anteriorly on the right. The left border is defined by the edge of the heart. Moving slightly inferiorly, the liver rapidly becomes larger, often extending from front to back. The left lobe is now seen anteriorly in place of the cardiac fossa. Usually no division between the right and left lobes can be seen at this level.

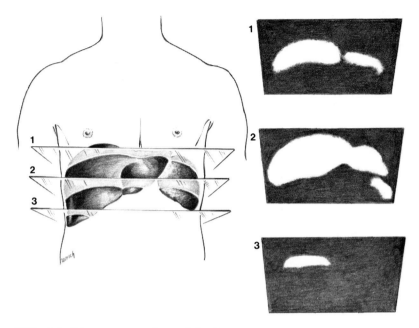

FIG. 6-5. Transverse sections of the liver.

In slightly lower sections, the separation of the liver into lobes becomes more apparent. First, there is a transverse separation between the left lobe and the caudate lobe, behind the left lobe and in front of the great vessels. There is then a vertical split between the right and left lobes, in the region of the ligamentum teres. At about this level, the right renal fossa may produce a concave indentation on the posterior aspect of the right lobe. The gallbladder fossa then appears on the medial side of the right lobe. Although there is considerable variability, the left lobe may end at about this level, and the right lobe continues down for a number of additional sections, occasionally ending as a long, thin, laterally placed strip called a Riedel's lobe.

The spleen, in the highest sections, may appear as an ovoid structure in the left posterior portion of the abdomen. The rounded posterolateral aspect fits smoothly to the body wall. In more inferior tomograms, the hilum appears on the anteromedial side, continuing down as a concavity. Small lobulations or completely separate accessory lobes may be present in the hilium.

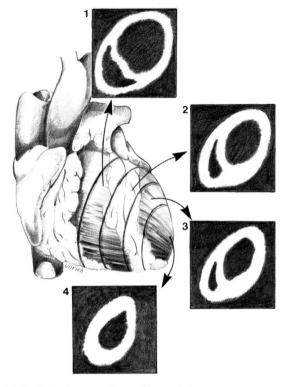

FIG. 6-6. Apex to base slices of the myocardium.

Thallium Myocardial Scan. The final example presented in this section is a thallium myocardial scan, sectioned obliquely from apex to base perpendicularly to the long axis of the heart (Fig. 6-6). The most anterior tomograms will show the apex, but the left ventricular cavity will become apparent as one sections more posteriorly. The activity will appear in a ring around it. It is now possible not only to assign names to the portions of the ventricular border (anterior, lateral, inferior, and septal) but also to predict the coronary artery that is most probably supplying each section.

If one orients the ring as though it were a clock, the region from approximately 7 to 10 o'clock is usually supplied by the main left anterior descending (LAD) coronary artery and its septal branches. The segment from 10 to 1 o'clock receives its blood from the diagonal (anterolateral) coronary branches of the LAD. The region from 1 to 4 o'clock is usually supplied by the obtuse marginal branch of the left circumflex artery (LCX), and from 4 to 5 o'clock by the posterior branches of the LCX. From 5 to 7 o'clock, the right coronary artery is usually the primary vessel. There is a good deal of variability, however.

CLINICAL APPLICATIONS

Bone

Recent surveys indicate that the bone scan is the most common in vivo nuclear medicine procedure in the United States. Therefore, if SPECT can increase the diagnostic efficacy of bone scanning, this one application of SPECT will have a significant impact on the practice of nuclear medicine.

The potential diagnostic advantage of SPECT lies in examining bony structures for which there is substantial underlying or overlying activity, which planar imaging techniques superimpose on the bony structures of medical interest. For example, in the hip, the acetabulum extends downward behind the femoral head. Therefore, the photon-deficient defect typical of avascular necrosis (AVN) of the femoral head may be obscured on the anterior planar view by activity originating in the underlying acetabulum. Using SPECT, however, it is possible to separate underlying and overlying distributions of activity into sequential tomographic images. For this reason, SPECT facilitates the detection of femoral head AVN.

Many bony structures suitable for SPECT imaging have not been studied in detail, and the potential of bone SPECT for oncologic imaging has not been thoroughly investigated. However, clinical experience to date has shown a role for bone SPECT in examining the knees, hips, lumbar spine, and temporomandibular joint (TMJ).

Bone SPECT has been found to be a sensitive noninvasive test for evaluating the extent of osteoarthritis of the knees. Differences in detection sensitivity for articular cartilage damage and synovitis were greatest in the patellofemoral compartment, where the sensitivity of bone SPECT compared favorably with the results of planar bone imaging, conventional radiography, and clinical examination. Furthermore, both SPECT and planar bone scanning are highly sensitive indicators of chronic tears of the meniscus.

Results suggest that bone scanning has potential as a high-sensitivity screening examination in patients with osteoarthritis or other significant internal derangement of the knee, particularly when augmented with SPECT.

Patients with clinical diagnosis of AVN of the femoral head have been examined by conventional radiography and bone scanning with SPECT. SPECT and planar bone scintigraphy are considered positive for AVN only if a photopenic bony defect can be identified. It has been concluded that when a photopenic defect is used as the scintigraphic criterion for AVN, SPECT bone scintigraphy is more sensitive than either planar imaging or radiography, not only when used at first complaints of hip pain, but also when symptoms have been present for as long as 18 mo. By identifying a photopenic defect that is not evident on planar views, SPECT can contribute to the accurate diagnosis of AVN of the femoral head.

In the past, planar bone scintigraphy was frequently incapable of distinguishing between increased metabolic activity in the posterior neural arch and underlying vertebral body of the lumbar spine. The value of this technique is thereby limiting as a means of differentiating between the various possible causes of low back pain and rendering correlation between sites of increased metabolic activity and radiographic findings less accurate. With the advent of SPECT, more accurate scintigraphic localization seems possible (Fig. 6-7).

Planar and SPECT bone scanning have been compared in adults with radiographic evidence of spondylolysis and/or spondylolisthesis of the lumbar spine. SPECT was more sensitive than planar imaging when used to identify symptomatic interarticularis. Furthermore, SPECT permits more accurate localization of abnormalities in the posterior neural arch. It has been concluded that when spondylolysis or spondylolisthesis is the cause of low

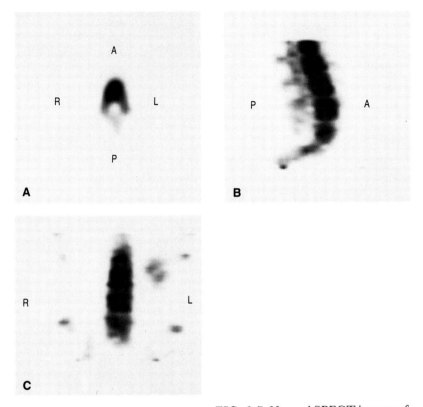

FIG. 6-7. Normal SPECT images of the lumbar spine. (**A**) Transverse. (**B**) Sagittal. (**C**) Coronal.

back pain, pars interarticularis defects frequently are associated with increased scintigraphic activity, which is best detected and localized by SPECT.

Planar bone scintigraphy has been shown to be superior to panoramic, transcranial, or tomographic radiography for detecting TMJ disease. However, arthrography rather than bone scintigraphy is commonly used to confirm the diagnosis of internal derangement of the TMJ, and bone scintigraphy has not previously been compared with the widely accepted arthographic standards for TMJ evaluation.

The diagnostic accuracy of conventional radiography, arthrography, and both SPECT and planar bone scanning has been evaluated in patients with TMJ dysfunction undergoing preoperative evaluation. The sensitivity of bone SPECT was comparable to arthrography and significantly better than planar bone scanning or transcranial lateral radiography. Compared with other imaging modalities, SPECT bone scintigraphy is the noninvasive imaging test of choice in screening for internal derangement of the TMJ.

For patients with knee, hip, low back, and TMJ pain, bone SPECT frequently gives images of greater clarity and in many instances provides unique diagnostic information. Specific advantages of SPECT in identifying and localizing skeletal pathology have already been established, and further diagnostic applications both for skeletal oncology and for the study of low back pain are anticipated.

Brain

Since Kuhl's first description of an analog backprojection technique, SPECT has been used for brain imaging. Some of the more recent efforts have concentrated on a comparison between SPECT and transmission CT. With standard radiotracers such as glucoheptonate or pertechnetate, good agreement was found between SPECT and CT for the detection of cerebrovascular disease; however, there was no clear-cut advantage to SPECT.

At approximately the same time, new agents were being described that promise to be useful for the imaging of cerebral blood flow. N-Isopropyl ^{123}I p-iodoamphetamine (IMP) was the first of these tracers to be described. The mechanism of cerebral trapping is still not clear, but it depends on the initial lipophilicity of the agent and on probable nonspecific intracellular binding. HIPDM, a diamine compound, also localizes initially proportional to cerebral blood flow, and its distribution and dosimetry are similar to those of IMP.

Cerebrovascular disease is the third most common cause of death in the United States, after heart disease and cancer. Until recently, nuclear medicine imaging of the brain in the evaluation of cerebrovascular disorders has been limited to compounds that only enter the brain where there is a disruption of the normal blood–brain barrier. With the advent of x-ray transmission CT, the use of traditional brain scintigraphy for the diagnosis of cerebrovascular disease has undergone a profound decline. The family of ^{123}I-labeled amines, however, readily crosses an intact blood–brain barrier and is retained by the cortex, providing new prospects to brain scintigraphy.

The distribution of these compounds in the brain reflects local cerebral blood flow. Regions of decreased or absent blood flow secondary to cerebrovascular disease appear as "cold" areas on the scintigraphic image. Changes in the pattern of the distribution of these iodinated amines occur early in the course of a cerebral infarction, well before a defect becomes apparent on the x-ray CT study (Figs. 6-8 through 6-10).

The discordance between CT and ^{123}I-IMP SPECT imaging is not surprising. The total extent of the stroke is likely to be quite different from the portion that is irreversibly damaged and becomes necrotic or highly edematous. Furthermore, metabolism and flow in pathways outside the zone of infarction may be affected by altered function within the stroke itself. In either case, it is likely that the ^{123}I amine study is depicting not only areas of infarction but also viable cerebral tissue that has decreased blood flow but sufficient metabolism to sustain the tissue. These findings would suggest that combined study of the patient with emission and transmission tomography may provide invaluable prognostic information concerning the extent of both reversibly and irreversibly damaged tissue.

Imaging with radiolabeled amines can also detect perfusion abnormalities in asymptomatic patients with normal CT studies but who have significant stenosis of the carotid or proximal cerebral

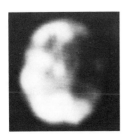

FIG. 6-8. Transaxial slice of brain demonstrating left cerebral infarction at onset of symptoms. (Courtesy of English RJ, Summerville D, Polak JF, *J Nucl Med Technol* 1984;12:13-15.)

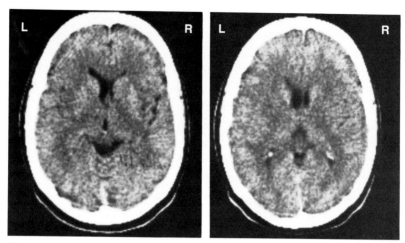

FIG. 6-9. CT scan performed 1 hr before SPECT, demonstrating no areas of infarction. (Courtesy of English RJ, Summerville D, Polak JF, *J Nucl Med Technol* 1984;12:13-15.)

arteries. Iodine-123 amine imaging appears particularly promising for follow-up evaluation of patients after surgical therapy. In limited studies of patients who underwent carotid artery endarterectomy for severe carotid stenosis, an improvement was shown in perfusion to previously abnormal zones after surgery (Fig. 6-11). Thus,

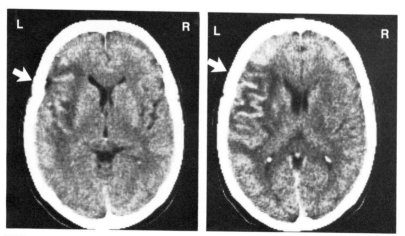

FIG. 6-10. CT scan 4 days postonset of symptoms producing region of infarct. (Courtesy of English RJ, Summerville D, Polak JF, *J Nucl Med Technol* 1984;12:13-15.)

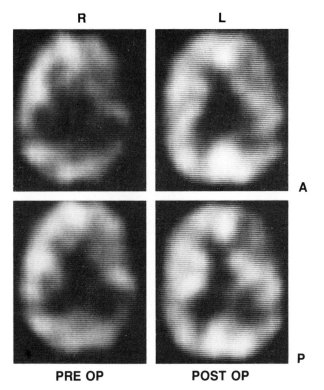

FIG. 6-11. Pre- and postendarcterectomy ^{123}I-HIPDM SPECT study demonstrating improved perfusion pattern.

perfusion imaging with ^{123}I amines may be useful in objectively documenting improvements in perfusion and possibly in assessing the complications of surgery as well.

Patients with dementia may pose particularly difficult diagnostic problems. Iodine-123-IMP imaging may be helpful in separating patients with Alzheimer's disease from those with multiple-infarct dementia. That is, multiple discrete asymmetric defects are seen in multiple-infarct dementia, whereas perfusion deficits in Alzheimer's disease tend to be symmetric and extensive (Figs. 6-12 and 6-13).

SPECT with radiolabeled amines is useful in a number of circumstances. First, in patients with acute cerebral infarction, the CT scan may be normal for several days after the onset of

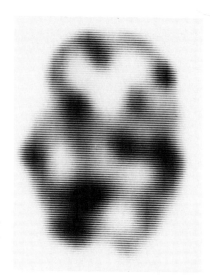

FIG. 6-12. Transaxial slices of ^{123}I-IMP perfusion in patient with multiple-infarct dementia.

symptoms, while the uptake of radiolabeled amines will be altered immediately after the onset of the stroke. Even when the CT scan has become abnormal, the physiologic abnormality may exceed the anatomic abnormality. Thus, SPECT may be able to measure the extent of the reversible ischemic tissue early enough to justify

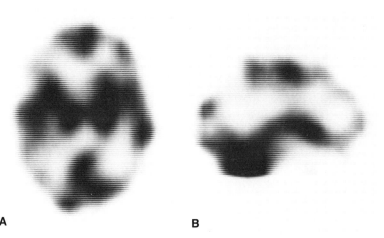

A   **B**

FIG. 6-13. (**A**) Transaxial and (**B**) sagittal slices of ^{123}I-IMP perfusion in a patient with Alzheimer's disease.

more aggressive therapeutic intervention. Second, medical and surgical therapies, such as endarterectomy, have been without readily available objective methods with which to access their efficacy. Serial measurements of regional cerebral perfusion with radiolabeled amines may provide such a tool. Third, in patients with epilepsy, the extent and location of the abnormally perfused focus may be important to medical and surgical management. Follow-up examinations may be useful in determining the effectiveness of therapy. Finally, the reliable diagnosis of multiple-infarct dementia as opposed to Alzheimer's disease could alter patient management and alleviate family concerns.

Gallium Scan

Gallium-67 has been used in the diagnosis of inflammatory lesions as well as neoplastic conditions, with variable degrees of success. Certain lymphomas and bronchogenic carcinomas are among the tumors that show particular avidity for gallium.

The role of ^{67}Ga scintigraphy in the management of patients with lymphoma has been controversial. Studies finding gallium scanning of limited value were commonly retrospective, assessing data from the late 1960s and early 1970s at a time when small doses (2–4 mCi) and outmoded technology (rectilinear scanners) were used.

The accuracy of gallium studies has been improved by the administration of larger doses of radionuclide (8–10 mCi) and the use of either dual- or triple-peak large-field-of-view Anger scintillation cameras. Recent studies have shown gallium scanning to be a viable tool in differentiating recurrent disease from bulky fibrosis following treatment, in both Hodgkin's and nonHodgkin's lymphoma. These studies recommended the use of gallium as an adjunct to chest radiography and transmission CT in following patients after therapy. However, optimal initial and posttherapy evaluation of patients with lymphoma requires not only the detection of disease, but also the extent and accurate localization of involvement.

Planar ^{67}Ga images suffer from a few constraints. Overlying bowel activity in the abdomen, and overlying activity in the ster-

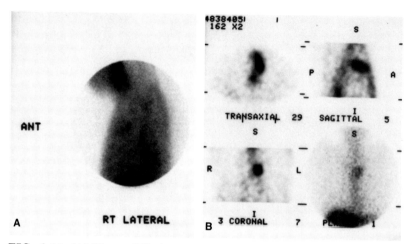

FIG. 6-14. (**A**) Planar ^{67}Ga images unable to detect mediastinal involvement and (**B**) SPECT images of same region.

num, spine, and in the mediastinum may interfere with thorough appreciation of the extent of disease, particularly when subtle residual uptake is to be depicted after therapy. Precise detection of anterior–posterior distribution is possible only with lateral views (Fig. 6-14). However, results are generally unsatisfactory because of attenuation and generalized poor target-to-background ratios. Planar images are generally unable to separate contiguous groups of involved lymph nodes, which may have a bearing on planning of treatment. For example, in a recent evaluation of 20 patients, planar images failed to differentiate hilar from mediastinal disease in two cases.

SPECT is a technology that has promising application in the management of patients with lymphoma. Transaxial slices provide not only improved sensitivity, but an additional plane of reference as well. Areas of increased gallium uptake within the mediastinum are easily localized in relationship to the sternum and spine. SPECT lends itself very effectively to the removal of this nontarget interference, providing a definitive map of ^{67}Ga activity, distributed between the sternum and spine, adding significant data to planar scintigraphic imaging of the chest. Moreover, the addition of SPECT is easily incorporated into the standard gallium imaging protocol.

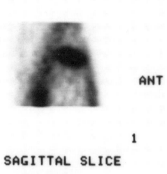

ANT

1

SAGITTAL SLICE
MID-CHEST

FIG. 6-15. Sagittal slices of ^{67}Ga distribution in mediastinal highlighting depth from sternum to spine.

Another unique aspect of SPECT imaging with gallium is the reorientation of the transaxial slices into sagittal and coronal planes. In instances of diffuse uptake, encompassing a large area behind the sternum, a more definitive map of the anterior-to-posterior distribution is presented. The depth and extent of an abnormality are easily visualized with both the sternum and spine present for reference (Fig. 6-15). In those cases in which the abnormality is immediately posterior to the sternum, a coronal slice provides an alternative method of separating gallium uptake in the sternum from that of the abnormal foci.

With its ability both to separate different foci of abnormal uptake from each other and from overlying normal tissue activity and to display images in transaxial, sagittal, and coronal planes, SPECT adds the dimension of depth that often separates the different abnormal nodal groups better than planar images (Fig.

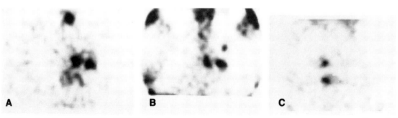

A　　　　　　B　　　　　　C

FIG. 6-16. SPECT of ^{67}Ga in chest demonstrating different abnormal nodal groups. (**A**) Transaxial. (**B**) Coronal. (**C**) Sagittal.

6-16). In addition, SPECT has shown foci of disease not clearly demonstrated on planar images (Fig. 6-17). SPECT might therefore be useful in the follow-up of patients with lymphoma, with a higher likelihood of detecting residual disease after treatment.

In many instances, however, the areas of gallium uptake are within the minimum range of detection and are surrounded with semiuniform background distribution. The lack or inappropriate application of uniformity correction (i.e., low statistic flood correction matrix) may generate a series of "hot" spots surrounded by concentric rings. In most cases, the center of the image matrix is the centroid of the thoracic cavity, producing a potential false-positive hot spot in the mediastinum. For the most part, these uniformity-correction artifacts are distinctive, requiring a great deal of imagination for misinterpretation (Fig. 6-18).

Studies using ^{67}Ga SPECT imaging in patients with lymphoma are under way, initially to define as many gallium-avid foci as possible, and then for follow-up evaluation with CT transmission or chest radiographs, which may provide a better estimate, due to the better spatial resolution, of bulk disease. When residual mass is noted, however, gallium SPECT is often helpful in differentiating residual disease from bulky fibrosis.

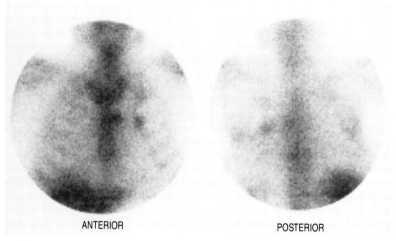

ANTERIOR   POSTERIOR

FIG. 6-17. Planar images of ^{67}Ga in chest, illustrating lack of clear presentation of foci.

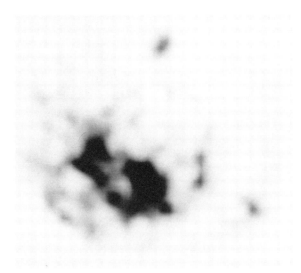

FIG. 6-18. Nonuniform correct transaxial slice of ^{67}Ga distribution in chest, illustrating characteristic ring pattern.

Liver

The use of SPECT in the liver has not been as thoroughly investigated as in the heart or brain. However, one proven use of SPECT in liver disease has been the measurement of liver volume. A number of groups have found good agreement between volume measurements made with SPECT and with liver phantoms; should liver volume estimates become clinically important, the technique has been well validated.

Of more importance is whether or not SPECT is useful in the assessment of hepatic metastases. Early indications are that there is higher sensitivity, specificity, and accuracy with SPECT than with planar techniques. Although sensitivity is poor with lesions below 2 cm, the high contrast of the image makes the technique superior to planar imaging in populations of low disease prevalence.

Cavernous hemangiomas are the most common benign tumors of the liver. Although their clinical course is usually uncomplicated, an accurate diagnosis may be important to exclude

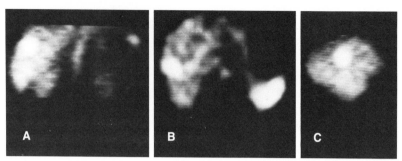

FIG. 6-19. SPECT images of ^{99m}Tc-labeled erythrocytes demonstrating deep-seated cavernous hemangioma.

risky percutaneous biopsy. Blood-pool scintigraphy is a reliable examination for the diagnosis of liver hemangiomas, but it may miss small deep-seated lesions.

The differentiation of cavernous hemangiomas from other space-occupying lesions in the liver is not possible by sulfur colloid planar scintigraphy or sonography. Computed tomography transmission is more specific. Cavernous hemangiomas appear as lucent lesions that are enhanced in a centripetal fashion. Although these signs do seem to occur with other lesions such as hepatomas and some metastases, blood-pool scintigraphy is reliable in detecting liver cavernous hemangiomas. There seems to be some controversy about the significance of the flow phase of the study, but most investigators agree that hemangiomas show a characteristic gradual accumulation of radioactivity. Two subgroups are difficult to detect. First, hemangiomas associated with extensive fibrosis, which replaces the cavernous component of the lesion, may not show the characteristic "pooling" of radioactivity. Second, small deep-seated lesions may fail to appear on the planar images because of the spatial resolution and overlying radioactivity. SPECT demonstrated improved detection of cavernous hemangiomas in this second group because of better separation of the lesion from overlying activity (Fig. 6-19).

Heart

SPECT was quickly found advantageous in imaging the heart. Many of the problems associated with conventional scintigraphy, such as superimposition of one portion of myocardium on another and the heterogeneity of background activities, are overcome with tomography. Imaging can be performed in planes parallel and perpendicular to the long axis of the left ventricle, thereby reducing interpretive errors caused by reduced perfusion at the base of the heart in the region of the valve plane.

Myocardial perfusion transaxial tomography has a characteristic appearance in the normal heart (Fig. 6-20). The left ventricle appears horseshoe shaped at the base of the heart, with the long axis of the horseshoe oriented between 35° and 45° toward the left anterior oblique. The distribution throughout the septum, anterior walls, and lateral wall of the left ventricle is homogeneous. The open end of the horseshoe corresponds anatomically to the aortic valve. Sections obtained at the mid-ventricular plane appear doughnut shaped, with uniform uptake throughout the doughnut. The central perfusion defect represents the left ventricular cavity. Slices through the apex show a round or oval region of activity with a minimal or absent central defect corresponding

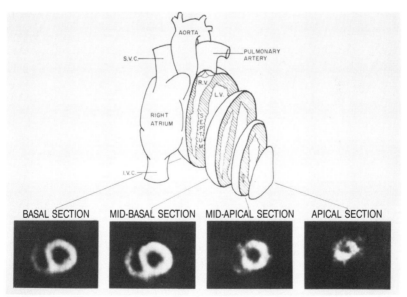

FIG. 6-20. Characteristic distribution of ^{201}Tl in SPECT imaging of the heart. (Courtesy of Kirch DL, Vogel RA, Lefree MT, et al. *Single Photon Emission Computer Tomography and Other Selected Topics.* New York: The Society of Nuclear Medicine, 1980.)

to a transverse section through the apical wall caudal to the cardiac chamber. Right ventricular or atrial activity is usually not detected. The left ventricle appears doughnut shaped in most images along the short axis (cucumber) plane.

In patients with myocardial infarction, regions of markedly reduced perfusion are seen in areas corresponding to the location of the infarct (Fig. 6-21). The extent of the perfusion defect is usually greater on emission tomography than on standard two-dimensional scintigraphy. Similarly, the border between the normally perfused myocardium and the perfusion defect is sharper and more clearly defined on tomography, since perfused myocardium is not superimposed on the ischemic tissue as it is with conventional imaging. Tomography also improves the contrast between the myocardium and surrounding structures, such as the lungs and liver. In addition to the improved accuracy over conventional two-dimensional imaging, the ability to obtain multiple transaxial slices of myocardial perfusion suggests the potential for volumetric quantitation of infarction or ischemia.

Tomography has been compared with planar imaging in the investigation of ischemic heart disease. Investigators have demonstrated, using ^{201}Tl at rest, that there is significantly higher sensitivity in detecting remote myocardial infarction with tomography than with planar imaging and that the increase in accuracy with tomography was largely due to increased detection of true positive infarcts in the posterior wall.

More recent work has concentrated on the use of ^{201}Tl in volumetric infarct sizing. Tamaki et al. showed that the volume

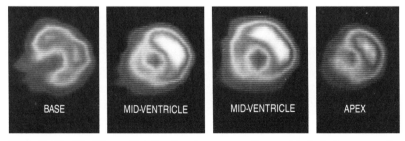

FIG. 6-21. Thallium distribution in myocardium with inferior–posterior infarct.

calculation of infarct size using SPECT correlated better with the degree of elevation in the MB isoenzyme of creatinine kinase (CK) in patients with infarction than from using mass by both SPECT and in vitro weighing, using a variable threshold to define boundaries. These investigators found good correlation between the SPECT and histologic measures of infarct size when using a threshold that varied with background activity. Maublant et al. demonstrated an excellent correlation between infarct size as measured by SPECT (using a manual selection of the infarct) and anatomic dissection. Thus, SPECT appears useful in measuring infarct size, whether with ^{201}Tl or with ^{99m}Tc-pyrophosphate, and with a wide range of data-processing protocols and instruments.

High-quality SPECT studies of the heart have recently been obtained with the introduction of a new class of ^{99m}Tc myocardial perfusion agents. Holman et al. (1982) reported that one of the hexakis(alkylisonitrile)technetium(1) cations, ^{99m}Tc(TBI), demonstrates viable myocardial uptake in both animals and humans. Photon yield from a 10-mCi dose of ^{99m}Tc(TBI) was an average of three times that of a 2-mCi dose of ^{201}Tl. This increased count rate permitted a 40%–50% reduction in SPECT acquisition times, with improved photopeak resolution. A ^{99m}Tc myocardial perfusion agent may change the current questions and conflicts regarding attenuation, 180° versus 360° rotation, and quantitation capabilities.

SUMMARY

After a long hiatus in the research areas of nuclear medicine, SPECT has begun to make clinical inroads. SPECT is fast becoming the imaging technology of choice in thallium studies and the undisputed method of demonstrating cerebral perfusion with radiolabeled amines. But the potential of SPECT does not end with just these studies. The complementary role of SPECT in such routine procedures as bone scintigraphy, gallium scanning, and liver imaging demonstrates that SPECT has a place in most clinical nuclear medicine settings. While investigators are continually reporting the promise and advantages of SPECT in specific conditions and abnormalities, the new user may find its greatest benefit as a technique to help resolve those "gray" ambiguous dilemmas of interpretation.

Throughout this text, a variety of techniques and possibilities have been described in an effort to acquaint the new user and refresh the experienced technologist with the diversity available in SPECT imaging. Whereas the fundamentals of SPECT acquisition, quality control, and imaging processing are for the most part standard, the clinical prospects remain open-ended, with new applications simply waiting to be implemented.

SUGGESTED READINGS

1. Anderson KC, Leonard RCF, Canellos CP, et al. High-dose gallium imaging in lymphoma. *Am J Med* 1983;75:327-31.

2. Carter BL, Morehead J, Wolpert SM, et al. *Cross-sectional Anatomy, Computed Tomography and Ultrasound Correlation.* New York: Appleton-Century-Crofts, 1977.

3. Collier DB, Carrera GF, Messer EJ, et al. Internal derangement of the temporomandibular joint: Detection by single photon emission computed tomography. *Radiology* 1983;149:557-61.

4. Collier DB, Johnson RP, Carrera GF, et al. Painful spondylolysis or spondylolisthesis studied by radiography and single photon emission computed tomography. *Radiology* 1985;154:207-11.

5. English RJ, Summerville D, Polack JF, et al. Brain imaging of cerebrovascular disease with I-123 HIPDM. *J Nucl Med Technol* 1984;12:13-15.

6. Holman BL, Hill TC, Magistretti PL. Imaging with emission computed tomography and radiolabeled amines. *Invest Radiol* 1982;17:206-15.

7. Holman BL, Hill TC, Polack JF. Cerebral perfusion imaging with iodine-123-labeled amines. *Arch Neurol* 1984;41:1060-63.

8. Piez CW, Holman BL. Single photon emission computed tomography. *Comp Radiol* 1985;9:201-11.

9. Royal HD, Hill TC, Holman BL. Clinical brain imaging with isopropyl-iodoamphetamine and SPECT. *Semin Nucl Med* 1985;-15:357-76.

10. Tumeh SS, English RJ, Holman BL. The complementary role of SPECT in the diagnosis of cavernous hemangioma of the liver. *Clin Nucl Med* 1985;10:884-86.

11. Turner DA, Fordham EW, Ali A, et al. Gallium-67 imaging in the management of Hodgkin's disease and other malignant lymphoma. *Semin Nucl Med* 1978;8:205-18.

STUDY QUESTIONS

1. *In tomographic images*
a. the spatial resolution is degraded.
b. presentation of structures are in an optimum relationship.
c. the reconstructed images are more susceptible to artifacts.
d. there is an increase in contrast between target-to-nontarget areas.
e. b and c.
f. all of the above.

2. *The projection images are created*
a. in a speed array.
b. in a narrow plane at right angles to the camera in transverse cuts.
c. at the same time the coronal slices are made.
d. first and then can be reconstructed into variously directed slices.
e. a and b.
f. b and d.

3. *In the conventional transverse cross-sectional presentation,*
a. the left side is on the left.
b. the right side is on the left.
c. a series should be presented from above down.
d. is viewed as though the patient is recumbent and seen from above down.
e. a and c.
f. b and c.

4. *In presentations of coronal sections,*
a. the right side is on the left.
b. the views are as though the patient is standing and seen from the back.
c. the front portion of the patient's body is on the top.
d. a and b.
e. a and c.
f. all of the above.

5. *A vertex view (planar) of the brain most closely resembles*
  a. a coronal section of a SPECT brain scan.
  b. a high transverse section of a SPECT brain scan.
  c. a projection coronal section of a SPECT brain scan.
  d. a low transverse section of a SPECT brain scan.
  e. a cranial tilt SPECT view.

6. *Oblique cucumber views are used in SPECT thallium images*
  a. because the heart lies at an angle in the body.
  b. to demonstrate the coronary branches.
  c. to section the heart apex to base perpendicular to the long axis.
  d. to better demonstrate the left ventricular cavity.
  e. a and c.
  f. a, c, and d.

7. *The xiphoid process of the sternum usually ends approximately*
  a. T4.
  b. T6.
  c. T8.
  d. T10.
  e. T12.
  f. none of the above.

8. *In a midplane section of the brain, you would be able to visualize anatomically*
  a. the tips of the temporal horns of the lateral ventricles.
  b. a separation of the frontal and parietal lobes.
  c. the brain stem.
  d. the cerebellum.
  e. a and b.
  f. b and c.

9. *Transaxial gallium slices of the thoracic cavity provide*
  a. overlap of counting statistics.
  b. improved sensitivity.
  c. an additional plane of reference.
  d. improved target-to-nontarget ratios.
  e. b, c, and d.
  f. all of the above.

10. *False-positive hot spots of gallium in the mediastinum surrounded by concentric rings can be caused by*
  a. gallium uptake just within the minimum range of detection.
  b. lack or inappropriate application of the uniformity correction.
  c. the extremely high concentration of gallium surrounded by low counts.
  d. bulky fibrosis residual disease.
  e. a, b, and c.
  f. all of the above.

11. *With a standard radiotracer* ^{99m}*Tc-GH, the comparison between SPECT and CT for the detection of cerebrovascular disease*

    a. proved SPECT superior to CT.

    b. showed no correlation.

    c. showed no clear-cut advantage of SPECT over CT.

    d. showed good correlation.

    e. a and d.

    f. c and d.

12. *SPECT* ^{123}*I-amine brain studies*

    a. can show altered distribution patterns early in the course of a cerebral infarction.

    b. can depict perfusion abnormalities in patients with significant stenosis of the carotid cerebral arteries.

    c. can differentiate patients with Alzheimer's disease from those with multiple-infarct dementia.

    d. a and b.

    e. a and c.

    f. all of the above.

13. *The left ventricle appears horseshoe shaped at the base of the heart in an oblique SPECT view; the open end of this horseshoe shape corresponds to*

    a. the mitral valve.

    b. the midventricle axis.

    c. the aortic valve.

    d. the septum.

    e. the right ventricle defect.

    f. none of the above.

14. *In thallium myocardial SPECT imaging,*

    a. no myocardium is superimposed over ischemic tissue.

    b. the extent of the defect is usually greater than that defect seen on the planar images.

    c. the border between normally perfused tissue and infarct is sharp.

    d. the contrast between the myocardium and surrounding organs is improved over that seen in planar images.

    e. a and d.

    f. all of the above.

PART II

INTRODUCTION

Chapters 1–6 of this text presented a general introduction of SPECT to the novice and a review of various protocols for the experienced. At this point, the new user may want to get started with patient studies while presenting an appearance of technical expertise. The veteran user, however, might be seeking greater flexibility or latitude in structuring existing protocols. In either case, SPECT presents an opportunity that is limited in technical and clinical scope only to the depth of the user's imagination.

In the remaining chapters, the procedures for a SPECT system's intital and routine evaluation and a few commonly imaged organ systems will be presented in a step-by-step fashion, providing the user with some semblance of a SPECT procedure manual. The examples are presented in a generic manner and are not meant to be taken as gospel or as an endorsement of any vendor's product or technique. They are offered only as the starting point that might be considered for individual expansion, suiting the user's unique needs. Each study contains examples of the author's concept of an acceptable transaxial slice, in addition to a number of flawed images of the same slice, with explanations of what went wrong. The reader is urged to use these clinically realistic images as a starting point for producing SPECT studies that meet the needs and criteria of the interpreting physician.

The first study presented is the newest and most exciting addition to SPECT, and by far the most technically difficult—the brain. A number of radiopharmaceuticals designed for brain perfusion studies are now or will be in the commercial market place. However, they present a host of imaging problems that may be resolved with a moderate amount of effort and a little patience. The brain is discussed first because those technical preparations and procedure tasks described for brain SPECT are also applicable and recommended for any other organ or SPECT study.

7 SPECT PERFORMANCE EVALUATION

The new user may well be overwhelmed by statements in the literature, or by manufacturers, regarding the complexity and temperament of SPECT imaging. As previously emphasized in this text, the technology of SPECT is not complex but is different and simply requires an open mind to get protocols successfully off the ground. If a system has been recently installed or is about to be finally utilized in a SPECT mode, it is recommended that a series of phantom studies be undertaken. These phantom exercises will serve three useful purposes: (1) orientate the new user with the instrument; (2) allay many misconceptions of SPECT's complex nature; and (3) provide a baseline set of an instrument's performance characteristics as a reference for future quality control purposes.

MATERIALS

Excessive costs need not be expended in the pursuit of routine quality control and performance testing. For all practical purposes, the only two items not routinely found in most nuclear medicine departments are the cylindrical phantom, with various inserts, and a refillable flood source. The bulk of items utilized for the procedures to be described should be available somewhere within any hospital.

By far the most useful tool for judging the noninvasive quality of a SPECT study is the 20-cm in diameter cylindrical phantom described in Chapter 3. Aside from its quality-control usefullness, the phantom provides an excellent source for hands-on SPECT education and experience. When loaded with some form of radioactivity and any number of available "hot" or "cold" inserts, the user is provided with some measurable spectrum for determining the cause and effect of various processing parameters through these experiments. The technologists, however, is not restricted to only those inserts that are supplied with the phantom. Home-made line sources and multisized geometric objects may be easily placed in the cylinder using masking tape and imagination. As each task is described, hints on phantom design will be provided.

The cylindrical phantom may be purchased with a number of inserts. These usually consist of a circular set of cold rods of varying diameters that are laid out like slices of pie. "Cold" rods are actually solid lengths of plastic that displace surrounding activity. "Hot" rods, on the other hand, are drilled holes of various diameters in a solid circular mass of plastic that are laid in various pie slice shapes. When immersed in activity, these rods fill, presenting lengths of activity in a nonradioactive background. A number of spherical, cold inserts also are available in different diameters. These objects appear as cold circular spots in an active background.

All the inserts mentioned fit very nicely into the cylindrical phantom. But a word of caution: practice setting up the phantom and its inserts in nonradioactive tap water. This will provide an opportunity to check for leaks and to get the feel of the fit and weight of the inserts. For instance, placing the hot rod inserts into nonactive water and then adding activity is not recommended by the authors. Proper mixing of the solution by shaking the cylinder does not always guarantee a homogeneous mixture, particularly in the smaller rods, and, in the long run, will mean prolonged, unneccessary exposure to the technologist.

The best solution we could recommend, is to load the cylinder half way with the required activity, stir with a long pipette, and gently submerge the hot and cold rod inserts. Watch for splashing and use plenty of absorbent paper and gloves. Again, practice on "cold" solutions first.

Line sources are easily created from butterfly tubing. Perfectionists might argue that extremely thin line sources, in the order of 1 mm in diameter, are required and that butterfly tubing does not meet this demand. In SPECT, however, the best possible resolution with a clinically designed rotating gamma camera is in the 10–15 mm FWHM range. Thus, even a 3- to 5-mm diameter tubing will not exceed the lower limits of most of the instruments on the market today.

Preparation of the line source simply requires attaching a syringe to the insert end of the butterfly tube, inserting the needle into a vial of relatively weak technetium-99m (^{99m}Tc), and withdrawing enough to fill the tubing. With a moderate amount of care, (be sure to use gloves and proper radiation safety techniques) tie knots on each far end, cut the tubing, and discard the syringe and needle. Attach the tubing to a glass or plastic pipette by stretching the tubing to a tight straight line and tape to the pipette. Thus, an inexpensive line source is ready for testing.

Another useful item for establishing SPECT performance capabilities is the 25-ml, 2-cm diameter scintillation vial. Disposable and inexpensive, these vials are available in glass or plastic and may be ordered from any of the laboratory products catalogs. They should also be readily available in most clinical laboratories. A number of experiments, outlined in this chapter make use of these simple accessories. For example, filling four of these vials with water, tapping to the exterior of the cold rod insert in a straight row, and submerging in as background activity of 250 μCi per ml within the cylinder will yield a projection set ready for reconstruction with varying filters and parameters. The user is thus provided with a set of four cold vials whose target-to-background ratios will vary with reconstruction factors and placement depth within the cylinder

ACQUISITION METHODS

The new user might find it helpful to conduct a number of basic phantom tasks prior to patient studies. These tasks will allow the user to become familiar with the system, while obtaining a number of useful parameters for future comparisions. For that matter, performing these protocols on a quarterly basis will provide the technologist with a complete, time-related record of the SPECT system's characteristics and behavior. The following procedures are

simply recommendations; users are encouraged to develop protocols that meet their needs, budgets, and time.

Center of Rotation

The first performance task conducted should be, and with a
number of commercially available instruments, must be, the center
of rotation (COR) acquisition process and correction factor install-
ment. With most systems, this simply requires placing a point
source in the immediate center of the rotational field of view and
following the manufacturer's protocol or recommendation for data
collection. In the most elementary terms, a drop of ^{99m}Tc (20–40
μCi) placed on the bottom of an empty needle cap, taped to the
end of a glass or plastic pipette, and secured to the end of the imaging table will suffice (Again, tape will do. Many of the great
phantom experiments of nuclear medicine would not be possible
without masking tape.) The protruding pipette assembly may then
be elevated and moved side to side, while monitoring the point
source on the persist scope, until it is within the center of scope
in both the anterior (0°) and lateral projections (90°). As
demonstrated, the need to purchase cobalt-57 (^{57}Co) point sources
is not necessarily warranted.

    Following the COR process, a photo of the COR graphs and
results should be taken and saved for future COR comparisons.
If the graphs are not smooth or do not meet the manufacturer's
guidelines, the process should be repeated once more while wat-
ching both the detector and the point source throughout the collection process for sudden or uncharacteristic motion. The vast
majority of poor COR collection and analysis can usually be attributed to an individual leaning on the imaging table or some other
outside force such as moving the point source during acquisition
(see Chapter 3).

Resolution

It is assumed that the buyer of a SPECT instrument has become
familiar with the resolving parameters of the gamma camera.
Measured in full width at half maximum (FWHM), most scin-

tillation cameras demonstrate FWHM in the order of 3–4 mm intrinsic and 5–6 mm extrinsic (LEAP collimator). It, therefore, often comes as somewhat of a surprise at just how poor the reconstructed resolution of SPECT may be. To determine this parameter, SPECT acquisition of a line source in air and in water is recommended.

Setting up the line source for air acquisition simply requires filling a butterfly tube with a moderate specific activity of ^{99m}Tc, stretching and taping to a pipette, and placing the apparatus within the rotational field of view. This may be either on the table or protuding from the end of the table, suspended in air. Placing the source on the table will provide the user with the effects of table attenuation, scatter, and the distance factor due to the required radius of rotation for table clearance. Suspension in midair will yield the truest uncompromised FWHM.

Collection parameters should be established that represent the highest possible resolution capabilities. For example, 128 frames collected in a 360-degree arc onto a 128 × 128 matrix will be well within the limits of a SPECT system's resolution (see Chapter 4). Acquisition time should be sufficient enough to reach one half the possible pixel overflow per frame.

To appreciate the effects of an attenuating material on resolution, one could repeat the procedure with the line source submerged in the center of a water-filled cylindrical phantom. This may be easily accomplished by installing the nylon center support bolt used to secure the inserts and taping the pipette with attached line source to this bolt. Fill the phantom with water, seal the top, place on the table, and collect with those parameters used for the acquisition of the line source in air. A word of caution when collecting SPECT data with the table in the rotational field of view: always manually rotate the detector under the table prior to data acquisition, to verify clearance, with either the phantom or patient in place. Many imaging tables will sag with the addition of a target's weight, requiring additional table elevation or detector adjustment for detector/table clearance.

Once acquisition has been completed, reconstruction will be necessary before analyzing the cross-sectioned line source. Two considerations must be given prior to selecting a filter/window combination. First, if sufficient counts/pixel were placed in the unreconstructed projection set, then reconstruction with a plain Ramp filter should suffice. Because there is no background activity, attenuation is not necessary. If, on the other hand, the counts/projection are not significant, some form of window will need to be multipied with the Ramp filter, to provide some suppression of noise. Should the user, for example, decide to apply a Ramp/Hann filter the selection of a cutoff frequency must take into account the acquisition matrix size. For example, a 64 × 64 matix might require a 0.5 rolloff. The same data collected on a 128 × 128 matrix would require a 0.25 rolloff to produce the same range of smoothing effect. Once both the line source in air and the line source in water are reconstructed into single cross-sectional slices, analysis for the FWHM may proceed (Fig. 7–1). If the reconstructed line source presents the appearence of a doughnut (Fig. 7–2), the COR collection process or correction factor should be suspect. With most SPECT systems, this will mean repeating the COR collection and phantom collection processes.

The first step in determining the FWHM is to place a profile through one of the reconstructed line sources (Fig. 7–3) to yield

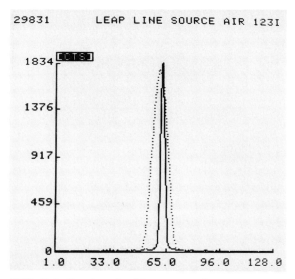

FIG. 7–1. Overlapping histograms of a reconstructed line source acquired in air (continuous line) and water (dotted line).

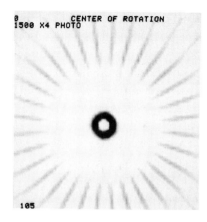

FIG. 7-2. Line sources reconstructed in a doughnut-shaped fashion due to improper COR correction.

a histogram (Fig. 7-3). The resultant curve then may be studied for the number of pixels separating the ascending slope at one half the maximum counts and also the descending slope at half the maximum. For example, if the counts at the peak of the curve were 2,000, then determination of the point or pixel on the *x* axis on

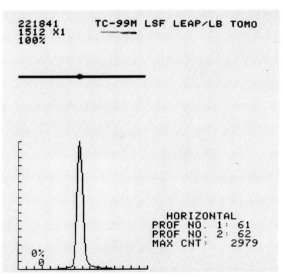

FIG. 7-3. To determine FWHM of a reconstructed line source, a histogram is placed through the reconstructed source (top) presenting a line spread response function (bottom).

each downward side is the 1,000 count mark. The number of pixel separations is the pixel FWHM. In millimeters, this could
roughly translate into the detector diameter in millimeters divided by the number of matrix pixels encompassing the detector field
of view. For example a 64 × 64 matrix covering a 40-mm diameter
detector would present a 6.2-mm distance for each pixel. A 128
× 128 would be reduced to ~ 3.1-mm/pixel. Thus a pixel FWHM
of 4 would roughly translate to 12.4-mm FWHM for a 128 × 128
matrix.

    This concept is not necessarily a realistic measurement. A
more exact method of measurement would involve setting up the
phantom with two line sources 10 cm apart before proceeding with
acquisition and reconstruction. A profile through both line sources
would present two curves (Fig. 7–4). The peak of each curve, or
maximum counts, would represent the center of each line source,
and the number of pixels separating these peaks would be equivalent
to 10 cm. For example, 30 pixels dividing the two peaks would

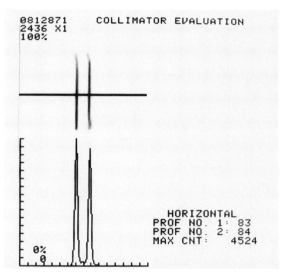

FIG. 7–4. Acquisition of two line sources with a
known spacing will yield two curves with related peak-
to-peak pixel distance. FWHM in millimeters may be
calculated by equating the known spacing with the
measured pixel distance.

be equal to 10 cm, or one pixel is equal to 3.3 mm. This would then be the conversion factor when converting FWHM in pixels to FWHM in millimeters.

Contrast

The ability of a system to distinguish objects of varying sizes and/or activity from its surrounding activity is known as contrast. Contrast is an important aspect of SPECT because the removal of over and underlying activity improves contrast. Thus, while resolution with SPECT is often at best poor, the improved enhancement of contrast redeems this imaging technique.

The following clinical situation offers a practical example: gallium scintigraphy in search of diseased para-aortic lymph nodes. Lymph nodes that may be diseased lie in a chain that travels just to each side and slightly anterior to the lumbar and thoracic vertebrae. If any one of these nodes or groups of nodes are disease-active, as might be expected in lymphoma, they will become gallium-avid. The problem encountered with standard planar gallium imaging is not one of resolution but the camouflaging of the nodes by the gallium-avid sternum, spine, left lobe of the liver, or soft-tissue activity in general. So planar imaging presents a situation of relatively adequate resolution but poor contrast due to over and underlying gallium-avid tissue. SPECT, on the other hand, peals back these layers of interference, isolating gallium-avid nodes, and removes the sternum or spine from the image. Granted, these nodes are not representative of the high resolution presented in CT, but how much resolution is really required to make a hot spot appear? Gallium SPECT imaging is discussed further in Chapter 10.

Thus, the new user to SPECT might be interested in performing some phantom experiments pertinent to examining the contrast capabilities of this imaging modality. If the phantom inserts are mounted with a bit of innovation, two sets of experiments may be collected with only one acquisition. Again, the 20-cm cylindrical phantom, six or seven scintillation vials, and the spherical inserts will play the major roles in this test.

The basic design of this phantom will be one of seven vials loaded with activity in concentrations that range from a 0:1 target-to-background ratio to a 6:1 ratio. Placed in a circular fashion, with the 0:1 vial in the center, a measure of the system's ability to present the activity and contrast of these vials in some form of a linear relationship will be sought. The circular spheres, provided with the phantom, will appear as cold objects of varying sizes in a hot background solution, providing the user with an index of the system's ability to distinguish contrast as a function of size. While the spheres come with attachments that allow for easy placement in the phantom, the vials will require the use of tape for a solid placement.

The first step in this experiment is to prepare the vials and background solution. The background solution should be sufficient to mimic clinical situations but not so great as to bring the system into the range of saturation. This will be a primary function of the phatom's volume. For example, most 20 cm diameter phantoms are long enough to hold approximately seven liters of liquid. A 1-μCi/ml concentration would require 7 mCi of total activity. In such a small volume concentration, this most likely would bring the detector close to the saturation point, possibly introducing a number of unfavorable variables that could influence the final image product not to mention the exposure produced by 7 mCi of unshielded ^{99m}Tc. Thus, the background activity could be prepared as 0.25 μCi/ml by mixing 1.75 mCi in seven liters of water. (This assumes, of course, that the phantom, with inserts, has a seven-liter volume.) Poor count rates can be adjusted and/or increased by simply collecting for longer or shorter periods of time. The background mixture may be prepared in the cylinder after the cold spheres have been mounted and set to one side.

To continue this phantom preparation, it is necessary to fill the scintillation vials with activities that range from 1:1 background solution to 6:1. This will require a modest amount of pipetting; however, the volumes are large enough so that the use of syringes will suffice. One method of vial preparation is to begin with a stock solution of ^{99m}Tc in a concentration of 1.5 μCi/ml (a 6:1 ratio with background) or 150 μCi in 100 ml. If 25 ml (37.5 μCi) are withdrawn and placed in a scintillation vial, the first vial of 6:1 activity is finished. This diminishes the stock solution to 112.5 μCi/75ml. Simply add 15 ml of water to the stock solution and a specific activity of 1.25 μCi/ml will be obtained. Withdraw 25 ml into the next vial and a 5:1 ratio is reached. This may be continued, using the instructions in Table 7-1, until all six vials are ready for insertion in the cylinder. A seventh vial, filled with inactive water, will serve as the 0:1 activity vial. These vials are then taped to the cold rod insert in a circular fashion, submerged in the cylinder, and placed in position for acquisition.

Acquisition can be conducted with either high resolution parameters or those that represent a more realistic clinical situation, or even both, depending on the user's desire to demonstrate the differences. Upon completion of data collection, the projection set should be corrected for uniformity variations and reconstructed with the manufacturer's recommendations for a sulfur colloid liver study. One vendor, for example, suggests a Ramp filter with Hann window at a 0.5 rolloff and an attenuation coefficient of 0.070. The rolloff is, of course, dependent on the matrix size and the counts collected. The greater the number of counts in the projection set, the sharper the cutoff. For example, 100K counts/projection might warrant a rolloff of 0.5, while 500K counts/projection might employ a 0.8 or 1.0 rolloff. If a 128 × 128 matrix is used, the rolloff point should be one half that of a 64 × 64 matrix. The slices selected should be those that include the hot vials and cold spheres.

Analysis of the transaxial slices would involve placement of

TABLE 7-1. Preparation of a Stock Solution of ^{99m}Tc for Filling 25-ml Vials in Concentrations of 0:1–6:1 Background Activity

Background Solution: 0.25 μCi/ml = 1.75 mCi/7 liters			
Stock Vial Solution	**Specific Activity**	**Volume Added**	**Ratio**
150 μCi/100 ml	1.5 μCi/ml	—	6:1
112.5 μCi/90 ml	1.25 μCi/ml	15	5:1
81.25 μCi/81.25 ml	1.0 μCi/ml	16.25 ml	4:1
56.25 μCi/75 ml	0.75 μCi/ml	25 ml	3:1
37.5 μCi/75 ml	0.50 μCi/ml	25 ml	2:1
25.0 μCi/100 ml	0.25 μCi/ml	50 ml	1:1
Water/25 ml	0.0 μCi/ml	—	0:1

regions of interest (ROIs) that are smaller than the reconstructed vials in their respective centers, and extracting the mean number of counts for each (Fig. 7–5). An additional ROI or ROIs also would be placed in areas of typical background activity (multiple background ROIs would be averaged to rule out random variations or fluctuations in counts). The contrast for each vial then could be calculated from the simple equation:

$$\frac{\text{target} - \text{background}}{\text{background}}.$$

An excercise of this nature would reveal a number of fundamental qualities regarding the SPECT system. First, by plotting the contrast of each vial as a function of the vial's specific activity (Fig. 7–6), the ability of the system to demonstrate some degree of linearity is documented. This graph also denotes at what

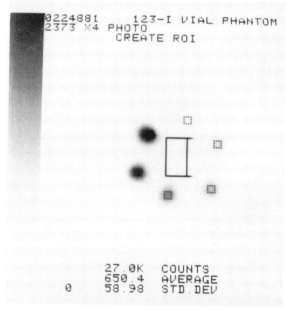

FIG. 7–5. Regions of interest (ROI) in vials centered from a transaxial projection set. Mean counts/ROI are extrapolated for analysis.

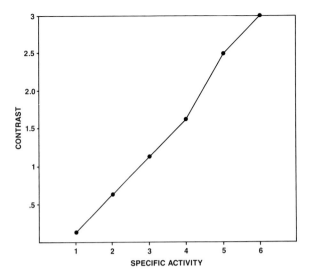

FIG. 7-6. A SPECT system's linearity is demonstrated by plotting the contrast of each vial (T-B/B) as a function of the vials specific activity.

point the system is able to distinguish hot activity from background. Plotting the contrast of the cold spheres as a function of diameter provides the user with some idea of the system's ability in resolving size. In both cases, the user also is presented with the opportunity to repeat the task with a variety of filter/window operations. As a learning exercise, a new user might reconstruct the phantom with a Ramp filter only, and a Ramp/Hann or Hamm, with a number of decreases in frequency rolloff. Aside from the visual changes, a greater shifting of the plots to the right on the x axis will be noted with each reduction in cutoff value. As expected, excessive smoothing will result in unacceptable image quality.

These phantom experiments are provided as teaching tools and are easily performed tasks for documenting relative contrast parameters. Users of SPECT seeking an absolute index for the testing of a system's contrast, signal-to-noise capabilities, or ideal reconstruction techniques should consult a physicist or search the literature for more advanced work in this area.

System Sensitivity

Although not a true measure of a SPECT system's reconstruction limits, sensitivity measurements are a useful method of
monitoring scintillation camera performance over a period of time
and are pretty simple to perform.

The measurement of the number of detected counts/unit of
source activity is an extrinsic test that evaluates the count rate performance of individual collimators. To conduct this test, one simply
needs to obtain a culture dish, or something of the same basic
design, and fill it with a known volume of water that almost covers
the bottom of the container. A large volume would be undesirable
since it would introduce attenuation and geometry as unknowns
and unnecessary variables. A thin film of solution on the bottom
will do nicely. A known amount of activity is placed in this volume,
mixed thoroughly, and placed gently on the inverted detector head.
Because these culture dishes do not seal tightly, be sure to place
a chuck or some form of highly absorbant paper on the detector.
Image the disk for a known period of time, record the number
of counts, and calculate the cps/μCi.

The user could, for example, prepare a stock solution of 50
μCi of ^{99m}Tc in 50 ml of water and pipette enough to cover the
base of the culture dish. This would provide a thin uniform distribution on a small portion of the detector's surface at 1 μCi/ml. The
dish is then imaged for 100 sec, yielding a total of, for example,
10,000 counts, or 100 cps. If the volume of activity covering the
bottom of the dish was recorded as 25 ml, then 100 counts/sec/25
ml divided by 25 μCi/ml would produce 4 cts/sec/μCi.

This technique is a relative one. However, if performed on
a quarterly basis, it will alert the user to any potential problems
involving sensitivity. While sensitivity is an indirect function of
SPECT, its stability is still important. One of the prime ingre-
dients of a quality SPECT image is an adequate information density (ID). If sensitivity degrades over time, longer collection times
will be required to provide an adequate ID.

Sensitivity Variations Versus Angulation

Variations as a function of the detector head's angle of acquisition should not result in sensitivity alterations. A test to verify this stability may be conducted by measuring a uniform, sealed ^{57}Co source, taped to the collimator face, and imaged at four consecutive 90° angles. A measure of count variations will provide an indication of the system's sensitivity as a function of angulation.

Positional Variations Versus Angulation

The integrity of the COR process, as well as the final reconstruction process, is dependent on a reproducible image, independent of the detector's acquisition angle. For example, a set of projection images to be reconstructed into transaxial images will depend on an entered COR factor for rotational alignment variation correction. Should the detector begin to slightly misplace detected counts on the collection matrix as the acquisition angle changes, then the proper application of COR correction factors will become unreliable, resulting in a modest to dramatic degradation of transaxial slice resolution.

A relatively simple method of montioring positional variations on a quarterly basis is performed by securely placing five point sources, of equal activity, on the collimator face in an appropriately spaced cross-fashion (Fig. 7–7) and collecting 32 projections over a 360-degree arc.

Four techniquess may be employed to analyze these data. The first and simplest way is to play back the projection set in a cine fashion and visually monitor the point sources for positional fluctuations. Remember that the point sources are attached to the collimator, thus, independent of outside positional influences, should show no movement at all. The second technique entails beginning the reconstruction process of the point source projection data and monitoring the sinogram image available on most systems. With five point sources, five uninterupted straight lines should appear. Breaks, or swerving in any one of the lines, may be indicative of positional variances and would require further investigation.

The third method of analysis is time-consuming and not always available as a software package. If available, the user could employ software that identifies the pixel occupying the individual point sources. By recording this pixel number as a function of the

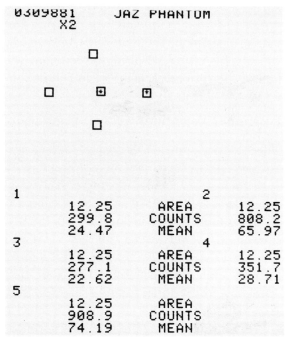

FIG. 7-7. Five point sources taped in a cross-fashion to the face of the collimator. The detector is initiated in a SPECT mode, and the point source activity is collected as a function of projection angle.

angle, a series of graphs could be produced revealing the positional changes of the point sources in the rotational collection circle. This is, however, a long and cumbersome project that may become more of an automated process like that described in the following technique.

The fourth technique requires the use of the ROI and curve generating software of the system's computer. If five small ROIs are placed in the center of each point source and the projection set is treated as a dynamic flow study, a set of curves may be generated, revealing the point source's shift as a function of acquisition angle (Fig. 7-8). This process virtually mimics the third technique but performs the task in a very short period of time with a minimum of effort by the user. The key to this technique is, again, to simply treat the projection set as a dynamic study.

Reconstructed Image Quality

The reconstructed slice is the final cross-section composite that results from a great deal of physical, mechanical, electronic, and mathematical interplay. As such, it could be considered as the last word in the performance testing process. The routine quarterly employment of a 20-cm cylindrical phantom for a pair of complete acquisitions will yield sets of transaxial images that will reflect one or any number of combinations of flaws in the SPECT system. These acquisitions should consist of the phantom with both the cold and hot inserts in place and a section with a uniform distribution of activity. Thus, the user is able to monitor uniformity, contrast, and resolution while also noting the total image quality that may or may not degrade with time.

The procedure simply may consist of preparing the phantom with its inserts and activity and collecting with both a high count set of collection parameters and a clinical set of collection factors. The image seen in Figure 7–9, is the cold rod section of

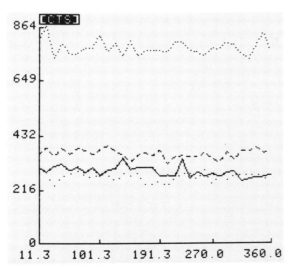

FIG. 7–8. Application of a curve generating program, as found in a dynamic flow analysis, plots the point source movement as a function of acquisition angle. The minor peaks and valleys are indicative of random noise in the counting process.

FIG. 7–9. Transaxial image of a cold rod section of a 20-cm diameter cylindrical phantom filled with ^{99m}Tc and collected onto a 128 × 128 matrix for a total of 128 projections for one million cts/projection. Projection data were reconstructed with a Ramp filter.

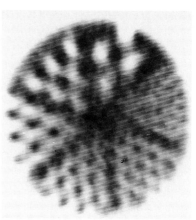

the phantom collected with a 128 × 128 matrix for 128 projections, with one million counts/projection, in an 11-cm radius of rotation. Figure 7–10 demonstrates the same slice of the same phantom, collected with a 64 × 64 matrix for 64 projections with 100,000 counts/projection, in a 20-cm radius of rotation. Both sets are reviewed with the previous quarter's set and saved for future comparisons. Reconstruction parameters (i.e., filter/window combinations) may vary with the user's concept of too little or too much

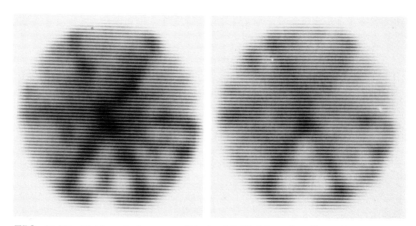

FIG. 7–10. Cold rod phantom filled with ^{99m}Tc and collected on a 64 × 64 matrix for 64 projections with clinically acquired statistics in the 100K cts/projection range. Projection data were reconstructed with a Ramp/Hann filter at a 0.5 roll off.

smoothing. The visual effects of various reconstruction parameters are demonstrated in Appendix G in the form of a cause and effect guide for the new user.

This test is not meant to be an absolute index of a SPECT system's characteristics, but it does represent a relatively simple method of monitoring a system's routine performance. If the images are of a consistent quality and nature, then the user may be relatively comfortable with the quality of the daily clinical studies. Should artifacts appear, which are not easily explained by poor uniformity or COR, then the user should use in caution in proceeding with further clinical studies until maintenance service has been scheduled.

SUMMARY

As described in this chapter, the bulk of SPECT performance testing does not require advanced degrees or outlandish expenditures. The technologist at a rural, 50-bed hospital is as capable as a physicist at a 1,000-bed university hospital in maintaining daily and quarterly performance testing procedures. The testing and analysis of resolution, contrast, sensitivity, and angular variations described in this chapter are easily conducted within any clinical setting with materials that are, for the most part, readily available in any medical institution.

It is hoped that the technologist confronted with a SPECT system for the first time will attempt these testing exercises as an introductory and familiarity process. Once the initial shock of a new technology is passed, the average user will find routine monitoring of a SPECT system to be only slightly more time-consuming, and certainly no more technically difficult, than the routine quality control of a dose calibrator.

SUGGESTED READINGS

1. Performance Measurements of Scintillation Cameras. National Electrical Manufacturers Association (NEMA). Washington, DC, 1986.
2. Murphy PH. Acceptance testing and quality control of gamma cameras, including SPECT. *J Nucl Med* 1987;28:1221–1227.

3. Raff U, Spitzer VM, Hendee WR. Practicality of NEMA performance specification measurement for user-based acceptance testing and routine quality assurance. *J Nucl Med* 1984;25:679–687.

4. Muehllehner G, Wake RH, Sano R. Standards for performance measurements in scintillation cameras. *J Nucl Med* 1981;22:72–77.

5. Hasegawa BH, Kirch DL. The measurement of a camera: Pathways for future understanding. *J Nucl Med* 1981;22:78–81.

6. Busemann-Sokole E, Cradduck TD. Interpretation of the NEMA protocols for scintillation camera performance. *J Nucl Med* 1983;24: 973–974.

7. English RJ, Zimmerman RE. Performance and acceptance testing of scintillation cameras for SPECT. *J Nucl Med Technol* 1988;16:132–138.

8. Croft BY. *Single Photon Emission Computed Tomography.* Chicago: Year Book Medical Publishers; 1986.

8 SPECT OF THE BRAIN

A large portion of nuclear medicine's history has revolved around imaging techniques for the brain. The first clinical tomograms of the brain using radiopharmaceuticals were produced by Kuhl, et al. in 1963. With the ready availability of technetium-99m (^{99m}Tc) and prior to the commercial explosion of computed tomography (CT), the ten years between 1965 and 1975 saw brain scintigraphy account for a great percentage of a nuclear medicine department's case load. However, because CT yields more specific anatomic information, and in many cases, better lesion detection, conventional radionuclide brain scintigraphy virtually disappeared from the scene.

Conventional brain imaging always has been misnamed. It is really nonbrain imaging, using radiopharmaceuticals that do not penetrate into the normal brain but will cross a damaged brain barrier and appear as focal areas of increased activity. This indirect method of brain imaging suffers from the constraints of poor structural resolution and minimal functional detail. This second item, functional detail, is of prime importance because a number of neurologic abnormalties occur with intact blood brain barriers and structural conditions. Positron emission tomography (PET) uses radiopharmaceuticals that readily cross the intact blood brain barrier, providing detailed functional mapping of the brain and allowing this imaging technology to resist the impact of CT and MRI and to remain at the forefront of neurophysiology and neurochemistry research. But PET is a costly technology and is presently limited to a few clinical sites, making it out of reach to the general clinical population. In the past few years, however, a number of single-photon emitting radiopharmaceuticals that also cross the intact blood brain barrier have made their way in the clinical nuclear medicine environment.

A number of these single-photon brain radiopharmaceuticals, ^{133}I-IMP, ^{99m}Tc-ECD, ^{99m}Tc-HM-PAO, are or will soon be commercially available, placing a very powerful clinical tool at the hands of the community hospital nuclear medicine practice. It remains, however, for the technologist and the physician to understand that the marriage of a technically advanced imaging modality, such as SPECT, with the complex structural and physiologic variants of the brain, provide for a number of unique technical considerations and hazards. While the problems encountered in perfusion brain SPECT may be found in SPECT of other organs, they are far more amplified in the brain. The remainder of this chapter is an effort to provide the new user of the iodine-123 (^{123}I) amine compounds and/or the ^{99m}Tc brain perfusion agents with the preliminary technical tasks and considerations necessary to produce quality SPECT images of cerebral perfusion.

The new user of SPECT and the brain perfusion agents should tackle six interrelated concepts, previously described in this text, as separate unique issues, that build to one final product. If each of these issues are properly addressed and handled, the final image product will be of the highest quality achievable, within the constraints or strengths of the instrument available. Those technical items that may make or break the goal of quality diagnostic brain slices are in order of performance: (1) collimation; (2) quality control; (3) patient positioning; (4) attenuation; (5) filtering, and (6) reorientation/display.

COLLIMATION

The necessity of proper collimation was addressed in Chapter 4, specifying a number of collimator designs specifically intended for brain SPECT. Unfortunately, the technologist given the task of producing a quality product is not always included in the process of purchasing the proper instrument or its accessories. Thus, in this and other cases, the technologist must make do with the available collimator. What is most commonly available in collimators for brain SPECT is what was delivered with the system, usually a medium-energy and an all-purpose low-energy collimator. However, even these two types fall into two groups—short bore and long bore. Representing the actual length of the hole from detector surface to collimator surface, the bore is usually a function of the collimator manufacturing process. Collimators manufactured in what is commonly called a foil or wafer process tend to have bore lengths on the order of 25 mm, while those produced with a cast process reach lengths of 40 mm. This extra length has an almost dramatic implication regarding the reduction of scatter photons reaching the crystal face, an issue of considerable importance when dealing with the high energy contaminants of [123]I. Aside from the problems of ^{123}I, the longer bore length, however, will mean reduced scatter for any radionuclide. Reduced scatter means reduced low-frequency amplification during the reconstruction process and, thus, increased contrast in the final image.

At this point, the technologist is faced with one of two collimator choices when collecting ^{123}I-labeled amine studies, the medium-energy or low-energy all-purpose collimator. If the collimator bore length is of the 25-mm type, the medium-energy collimator will prove the most effective in reducing the high energy breakthrough of the [124]I contaminant of [123]I. The low-energy all-purpose or even low-energy high-resolution foil designs simply do not place enough length of absorbing medium between the photon entrance to the collimator and crystal surface to significantly reduce scatter that will eventually be reconstructed as low frequency background. These short bore collimators are specifically designed to collect photons arising from the 140 keV photopeak of ^{99m}Tc in a planar mode and do not perform well at reducing scatter and improving contrast under SPECT conditions. This is, however, not quite as much of a problem with the 40-mm length cast-produced low-energy collimators, as demonstrated by Polack, et al. Their work demonstrated that with these designs sufficient lengths of absorber are present to reduce unwanted scatter, while at the same time retain resolution. If the SPECT system utilized is supplied with this style collimator, the choice of the low-energy all-purpose, or low-energy high-resolution collimator proves a better one than that of the medium-energy design.

Thus, once the user has established the bore length of the SPECT system's supplied collimators, the next step in the protocol design process may be taken. As previously noted, a number of innovative collimator approaches to brain acquisition were addressed in Chapter 4. The use of a long-bore, fan-beam, cone, and even slant-hole collimator provides either reduced target-to-detector distance and/or reduced scatter and thus improved contrast, while still retaining, and in some cases, improving resolution. It is unfortunate that these designs are not readily commercially available. One argument theorizes that improved radiopharmaceuticals possibly will make collimators unnecessary. This could not be farther from the truth because any of the conditions that provide for improvements with less than optimal radionuclides also will be passed onto the ^{99m}Tc radiopharmaceuticals. Figure 8–1 demonstrates the improvements in contrast between a ^{99m}Tc-ECD perfusion brain scan collected through a LEAP collimator and through a long-bore collimator. Should a user find a substantial demand for perfusion brain SPECT, the purchase of one of these specialty colli-

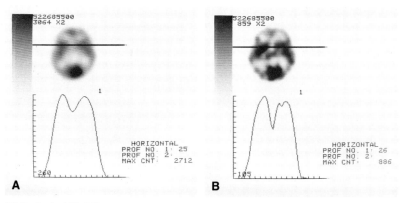

FIG. 8–1. (A) Histogram plotted through a ^{99m}Tc-ECD mid-brain transaxial slice collected with a 41-mm bore length LEAP collimator yielding a poor range of contrast. **(B)** Histogram through the same brain slice acquired through a 139-mm bore length "long bore" collimator, yielding considerable contrast improvement.

mators should receive a great deal of consideration.

Following collimator selection, the new user to brain perfusion SPECT should consider running through tasks number two through five, employing a series of phantom exercises prior to patient acquisition and processing. The phantom type mentioned in Chapter 3, filled with ~ 2–4 mCi of commercially available liquid ^{123}I, or perhaps even eventually ^{99m}Tc, will suffice for this procedure. The point to this task is to work out the bugs in positioning a patient within the constraints of the system's table and head holder, provide the user with those data necessary to establish attenuation correction coefficients, filter amplitudes and cutoffs, and to verify the quality-control integrity of the system. As would be expected, this last point, quality control, is of the utmost importance in brain SPECT for the simple reason that the vast majority of collected data resides in both a relatively homogeneous state and in a small count-compressed field of view. Hence, even marginal errors in the COR or uniformity correction will be substantially amplified.

QUALITY CONTROL

The image degradation caused by poor COR correction is amply demonstrated in Figures 8-2A and 8-2B. Figures 8-2A demonstrates

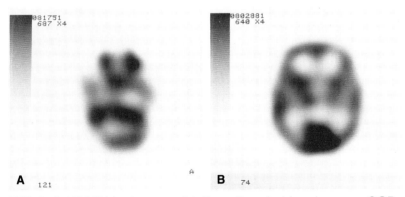

FIG. 8–2. (A) Mid-brain transaxial slice collected with an improper COR, presenting a smearing effect of the cross-sectional anatomy. **(B)** The same mid-brain slice reconstructed with a proper COR and resultant correct placement of structural anatomy on the image display matrix.

a transaxial, mid-brain slice collected with an improper COR, while Figure 8-2B shows the same slice with the properly applied COR. It must be remembered, that the COR process is not retrospectively applied on most commercial systems; hence, the 10- to 20-minute task of correct COR application should be done prior to the day's brain acquisition. This will save a multitude of problems with later processing and display. Figure 8-2A impressively demonstrates the smearing effect and image degradation that occurs when rotational misalignment is not properly corrected for with the COR process.

Figure 8-3A demonstrates a transaxial brain slice with the customary bull's-eye artifact generated as a result of poor uniformity correction, as described in Chapter 3. The properly corrected slice is shown in Figure 8-3B. The leading cause of poor uniformity correction with ^{123}I amine studies is the inability of most SPECT detector systems to properly accommodate the nonuniformities of [124]I contaminated [123]I. Simply put, the response of the photomultiplier tubes and resultant correction efforts for this radionuclide are not the same as those with [99m]Tc. Hence, the

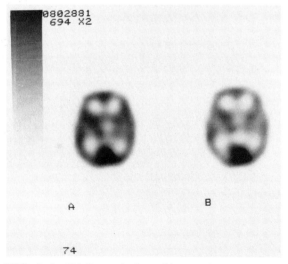

FIG. 8-3. (A) Degradation of internal structures in a mid-brain transaxial slice due to poor uniformity correction and (B) the same slice properly corrected, presenting a higher definition of internal structures.

uniformity correction of an ^{123}I-amine study with a [57]Co- or a ^{99m}Tc-flood source will yield less than optimal results, as demonstrated in Figure 8-3C. The user who plans to collect ^{123}I amine brain scans on a weekly basis should consider purchasing one of the refillable sources mentioned in Chapter 3 and loading it with an inexpensive amount of liquid [123]I (1 mCi is sufficient for a 30–60-million count) overnight or at least bimonthly for flood collection.

With the completion of these quality control necessities, collection of a phantom, and eventually the patient, may begin. The phantom is usually in the order of 20 cm in diameter with an average of seven liters for volume, depending on the number of inserts. To simulate the brain uptake of a perfusion radiopharmaceutical, a concentration of 1 μCi/ml might be considered physiologically realistic, but for practical purposes it is photonexcessive in a phantom. Even if the phantom is loaded with all of its hot and cold inserts, roughly 4–5 mCi of the radionuclide will be required to reach this concentration. This poses two problems. First, it is expensive, and secondly the excess volume and resultant activity will saturate the detector. Therefore, an acceptable phantom procedure might involve loading a dose of 0.25–0.4 mCi/ml into the container with both the hot and cold rods in place. One section should be void of inserts in order to be used for the evaluation of uniformity and the determination of attenuation coefficients.

PATIENT POSITIONING

The cylinder may now be placed in the head holder, and the detector may be positioned in such a way that placement best simulates actual patient acquisition. This will probably involve a radius of rotation in the order of 15–17 cm. Collection parameters should be established that realistically simulate patient acquisition. This would imply a collection of at least a total of three million counts for the complete 64 projections, or in a "step and shoot" mode, ~ 50,000 counts/projection. This is what typically might be expected as a count rate for a normal patient receiving a 3–5-mCi administration of ^{123}I iodoamphetamine. It is necesary when collecting the phantom data, that the time of acquisition be adjusted to produce this count rate so that realistic patient equivalent data are produced for evaluation of reconstruction filter/window combinations.

The following notes are applicable for both patient and detector head positioning:

1. Always center the target in the field of view with four different angled views using the persist scope or positioning mode prior to data acquisition, especially if a 1.5-zoom mode is employed. The patient who is perfectly positioned and centered in the anterior position may be 2 cm out of the field of view in each of the lateral projections, requiring a height adjustment to the table.

2. Always rotate the detector around the patient at least once for safety reasons. In an effort to reduce target-to-detector distance, a user may end up scraping the underside of the table or possibly injuring a patient's shoulder if care is not taken.

ATTENUATION CORRECTION

All commercially available SPECT systems supply some method of attenuation correction, whether it be the "Sorenson," "Chang," or simply some manufacturer's variation. While the merits of these techniques supply a great deal of debate, the need for some type of attenuation correction for perfusion brain SPECT with either ^{123}I or ^{99m}Tc appears necessary. The lack of some form of attenuation correction application will produce images with high intensity edges and almost nonexistent internal structures (Fig. 8-4A). Therefore, the determination of an attenuation coefficient for ^{123}I becomes a must, prior to patient data reconstruction, to provide cross-sections of the brain that attempt to be realistically indicative of brain anatomy (Fig. 8-4B).

Before describing the techniques of determining the attenuation and reconstruction parameters that may be employed by first time users of brain SPECT, a word of caution and an apology to the physicists and experts of nuclear medicine in general and SPECT in particular are offered. The techniques to be described

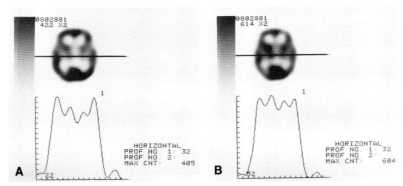

FIG. 8-4. (A) Histogram plotted through mid-brain slice reconstructed without attenuation corrrection, demonstrating increased activity on the edges and reduced anatomic definition of the internal structures. **(B)** The same brain slice corrected for attenuation showing a uniform count intensity across the histogram.

are a shotgun approach to some complicated problems. They are not by any stretch of the imagination absolute and are only presented as starting blocks for the SPECT beginner.

In order to identify the proper cutoff frequency for a particular filter/window combination to be used with ^{123}I and some new collimator design, a physicist might collect and analyze a series of line sources collected through this collimator. The data from the line spread functions might then be used to generate the modulation transfer function (MTF) of that particular radionuclide unique to that individual collimator. The rolloff that these data yield then would be used to determine the amplitude and frequency cutoff of the particular filter/window combination in question. This method of data analysis is useful, but it usually requires software not available with most commercial SPECT systems. The following suggestions are shortcut approaches to producing minimally acceptable processing parameters that may be performed with any system to provide diagnostic images.

As explained in Chapter 2, the immediate effect of a noncorrected uniform distribution of radionuclide in a cylinder is a transaxial image with sharp, high-count intensity edges that theoretically decrease expoaentially toward the center. The goal of properly applied attenuation correction is to produce a transaxial slice of a uniform source, whose counts/pixel in the center are anatomically proportional to the edges.

Having completed SPECT acquisition of the ^{123}I filled phantom, the user should then correct for uniformity variations with the 30–60 million count flood previously described. The uniform distribution region of the phantom (that area not containing hot or cold rods) is then selected for reconstruction, using the individual system's method of slice selection. The user then introduces some basic reconstruction parameters (i.e., Ramp-Hann filter with a 0.5 rolloff) but does not at this point introduce an attenuation correction factor. This will produce a baseline slice with the sharp edges just described. The placement of a profile through the slice will demonstrate the degree of amplification required to produce uniform distributions (Fig. 8–5A).

A number of commercial systems allow the user three options during the reconstruction phase for attenuation correction: (a) not to apply it at all; (b) use the manufacturer's coefficients; or (c) introduce coefficients of ones own choosing. The latter will be applied for this present effort. The user should, at this point, simply repeat the single slice reconstruction process with the application of some coefficient that will raise the bow in the profile of Figure 8–5A. Figure 8–5B, for example, demonstrates the effects of a coefficient, $(\mu) = 0.020$. This process is repeated, or iterated, until a flat profile develops (Fig. 8–5C in which $\mu = 0.030$; and Fig. 8–5D in which $\mu = 0.040$). The coefficient that provides this flat profile is then applied for all future patient studies.

FILTERING

As presented in Chapter 5, filters and windows are the tools that supress background and, hopefully, reduce noise. The degree of smoothing produced by this function is for the most part a matter of individual taste, covering a spectrum that goes from the very smooth, suppressing any detail, to the coarseness of gravel, which masks and hides data. However, one of the nice things about filter functions is that they generally are performed retrospectively, allowing the user the option of attempting any number of combinations without imposing on the patient's time or health status. There

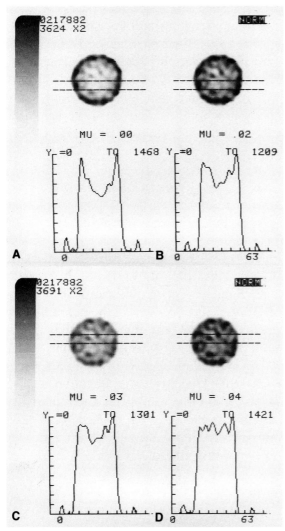

FIG. 8–5. Histogram plotted through a reconstructed cross-section of a uniformly filled phantom with an attenuation correction coefficient (μ) equal to **(A)** 0, **(B)** 0.02, **(C)** 0.03, and **(D)** 0.04. Each increase in the value of μ raises the bow in the histogram.

are, however, some simple phantom exercises that might provide the new user with a comfortable starting framework prior to actual patient applications. These phantom projects may be particularly useful if the study to be performed, such as brain perfusion SPECT, present unfamiliar anatomic structure and appearance.

Some of the high bandpass filters such as the Butterworth, when not applied correctly, may amplify discrete heterogeneous areas into noticable hot spots that may not actually exist. Other filters, such as the Hann or Hamm may look pretty but might very well be limiting or smoothing together the full potential of raw data collected by the detector. Determining an ideal filter/window combination that is clinically useful is at best a difficult task and at worst is the source of a great deal of debate. The following procedure, however, is one ballpark method of justifying the selection of a filter/window function for brain perfusion studies when the expertise of a physicist or engineer is not available.

Prepare the 20-cm diameter phantom with a homogenous volume of the radionuclide to be employed, ^{123}I or ^{99m}Tc, in a concentration of 0.25 mCi/ml (This will be the background activity.). Prepare six 25-ml, 2-cm diameter vials (liquid scintillation counting vials will do nicely) with concentrations of the radionnuclide in ratios of 1:1, 2:1, 3:1, 4:1, 5:1, and 6:1 to background as well as a seventh vial with nonradioactive water. Tape these vials on the outer edge of either the cold rod or hot rod insert in a circular fashion and place them into the 20-cm cylinder. Phantom acquisition should be performed with those conditions and parameters used with patients. Upon completion of data collection, correct the raw data for uniformity variations and reconstruct a slice using the manufacturer's recommendations if available.

The reconstructed cross section of the phantom should present itself as some variation of Figure 8–6, with a number of the vials appearing in the circular array. Data are now available to evaluate for sensitivity, linearity, contrast, and signal-to-noise ratios. These factors may be calculated from ROI software, available with most commercial packages (Fig. 8–7), and used as a crude quality index for determining the best, or at least better, reconstruction parameters.

For instance, the vial activity demonstrated in Figure 8–6 was retrieved from a slice reconstructed with a Ramp-Hann filter, with a 0.5 rolloff, and yielded the data listed in Table 8–1 (The same slice was reconstructed with a straight Ramp filter, a Butterworth,

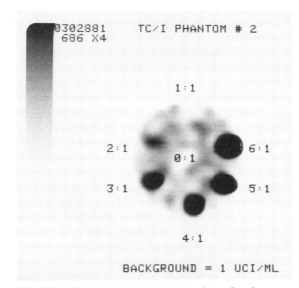

FIG. 8–6. Reconstructed cross section of a phantom containing seven vials of activity in ratios of 0:1 to 6:1 to a background activity of 1 μCi/ml.

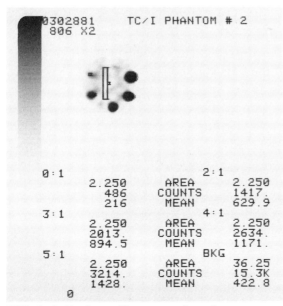

FIG. 8–7. Regions of interest and resultant extrapolated data from the phantom described in Figure 8–6.

TABLE 8–1. Effects of Filtering

	Ramp		
Vial	Mean Counts	T-B/B	T-B/SD
0	152	−0.64	−8.6
1	427	0.01	0.1
2	694	0.64	4.0
3	935	1.22	5.9
4	1259	1.98	6.6
5	1514	2.59	5.8
6	2021	3.79	12.5
Bkg	422		
	Ramp/Hann (0.25)		
0	355	−0.18	−13.9
1	409	−0.06	−0.15
2	568	0.31	19.8
3	659	0.52	15.8
4	748	0.73	27.6
5	866	1.00	19.6
6	1142	1.63	29.8
Bkg	433		

and a Ramp-Hann with a 0.25 rolloff.). Simply plotting the mean number of counts/vial as a function of each vial's activity yields both the linearity of the process and the lowest possible detectability of activity for any of the four applied filter functions (Fig. 8–8). Carrying the process further, contrast is determined by subtracting the background from the mean counts of each vial, dividing by the background, and plotting the results as a function of vial activity (Fig. 8–9).

While this process may seem complicated, it realistically occupies only a couple of days worth of work and does provide a simple lab experiment that demonstrates the effects of filtering. For instance, if the counts versus activity in Figure 8–8 is studied, it is apparent that filtering of any type supresses image counts (Table 8–1). The Ramp filter results in virtually no smoothing operations but retains the best linearity, while inducing very little influence on counts. At the other extreme, the Ramp-Hann with a 0.25 cutoff manipulates the counts, reducing them by almost half, while also altering the linear relationship of the vial's activity. The user has

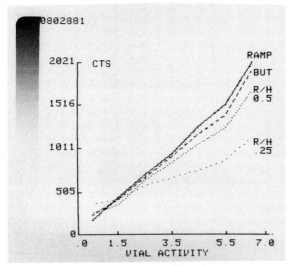

FIG. 8–8. Graphic demonstration of count suppression caused by increased rolloff of a Hann filter function. Counts extrapolated from activity vials are reduced and lose linearity as the rolloff factor is reduced.

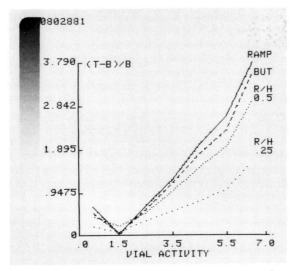

FIG. 8–9. Reconstructed vial contrast, measured as the absolute value of target activity minus background, divided by background, versus vial activity becomes degraded as the filter rolloff factor is reduced, altering structural detectability.

to keep in mind, however, that the Ramp filter by itself is too noisy and literally uninterpretable for low-count clinical studies. Thus, some smoothing or window function is needed, and the Butterworth filter, in this example, seems to come closest to retaining those properties of the Ramp filter while avoiding the overdone smoothing of the Hann window.

Figure 8–9 presents the idea that either the Butterworth or Hann, with a 0.5 cutoff, comes closest to the Ramp in retaining contrast. Again, while the Ramp is quantitatively the best, its total lack of smoothing makes it useless for practical work. The need to apply some form of smoothing is apparent but the question of how much or when to stop is always present. The problem with this example, however, is that the extreme cutoff of 0.25 eliminates useful image data as well as noise. Again, the Butterworth and Ramp-Hann with a 0.5 cutoff applies a moderate degree of noise reduction without severely degrading the target's useful data.

Although this process may seem somewhat complicated to a new user who simply wants to get started, proper filter/window combinations, as demonstrated in Figure 8–10, can turn a poor diagnostic image into one of publishable quality. Figure 8–10A demonstrates the noisy "salt and pepper" appearance of a transaxial brain slice when only the Ramp filter is employed. A profile is placed through the right and left striated cortex with the resultant histogram revealing some degree of separation between the two sides. The Ramp-Hann filters generally degrade the contrast, while the Butterworth filter tends to reveal the sharpest definition. The question regarding which filter should be employed initially for brain perfusion SPECT is best answered by the user's results from trial and error processes because each SPECT system will respond differently to the uniqueness of the brain perfusion agents.

DATA DISPLAY

As mentioned in Chapter 5, final image production does not end with the transaxial images. As nuclear medicine specialists become more familiar with perfusion brain SPECT, the amount of information available in coronal and sagittal sections increases. Recog-

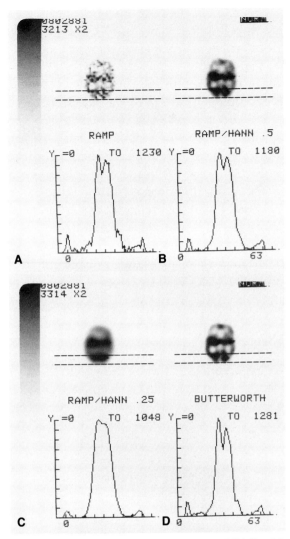

FIG. 8–10. Transaxial slices of ^{99m}Tc-HM-PAO mid-brain study demonstrating the **(A)** excessive noise generated by a Ramp filter, **(B)** the moderate smoothing of a Ramp/Hann filter with a 0.5 rolloff, **(C)** the over smoothing of a Ramp/Hann filter with a 0.25 cutoff, and **(D)** the improved structural separation produced with a Butterworth filter. Histograms are plotted through the striated region of the brain, presenting the ability of a correct filter to separate activity between two hemispheres.

nized as one of the advantages of the rotating gamma camera as opposed to the single slice systems, including PET, is its ability to produce volumetric information or images that present the organ of study as a whole (Fig. 8–11).

All commercially available rotating gamma cameras provide a coronal/sagittal generating software package that functions in a rather basic manner. The complete set of transaxial images are simply stacked on one another to form a sort of matrix cube, and the coronal or sagittal images are extracted from the front or from the side of this cube (see Chapter 5). Thus, an area of interest or a defect may be isolated and pinpointed for further study (Fig. 8–12). Most SPECT systems allow the technologist or physician to sit at the display console and thumb through these slices in an orderly fashion. There are, however, three issues related to the brain that the user should consider when reviewing or displaying these data: (1) partial volume effects; (2) positional inconsistencies; and (3) single slice limitations.

Partial Volume Effects

Partial volume effects are an intrinsic flaw of the system that cannot be avoided. To better understand this concept, consider the

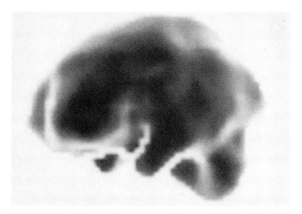

FIG. 8–11. Composite image of processed transaxial slices stacked together using a technique known as distance weighted reprojection. This software technique allows the user to rotate the brain on an axis and view the structure as a total volumetric entity.

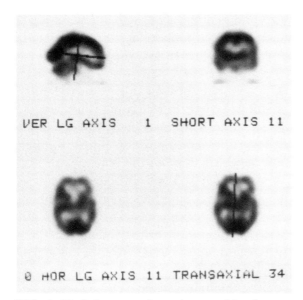

FIG. 8–12. Software package that provides the user
with the ability to view three planes on the same screen
and pinpoint a defect with cross hairs.

collection and reconstruction of a line source, whose length en-
compasses three pixels. The resultant data might be displayed as
three cross-sectional slices respresentative of each row of pixels containing data. A histogram placed through each line source cross
section would, in effect, present a line source response function
in the x and y directions. If one imagined the same profile applied
in the z direction, or the slice-to-slice relationship and the distance
between peak activity indicative of true slice-to-slice distance, one
would observe a great deal of overlapping information at the lower
portions of the curves. The shaded areas unde the curves represent the amount of information that spills over a slice of interest
from its two ajoinging neighors. Thus, the study's slice also is
representative to some degree of neighboring slices.

Positional Inconsistencies

The second consideration when interpreting perfusion brain studies
is the potential of positional inconsistencies. It is realistic to assume

that many patients who undergo this study are unable to easily maintain a classic straight anatomic position for the required study time. Patients who have suffered strokes or who might have advanced osteoporosis tend to be comfortable in the head holders only when their head may be rotated or their chin elevated. It often is better to acquire the study in these imperfect positions with the patient's cooperation than risk constant movement throughout the exam. Should the patient not be ideally positioned, the user has, in most cases, the ability to straighten out the images with software at a later time. Most SPECT software packages contain an oblique reorientation program, usually designed for thallium studies, that work effectively with brain studies. Figure 8–13A demonstrates the reconstructed brain slice of an individual whose head was significantly hyperextended and whose chin was hyperextended, resulting in a brain slice with very little anatomical symmetry. With this particular thallium software package, the user

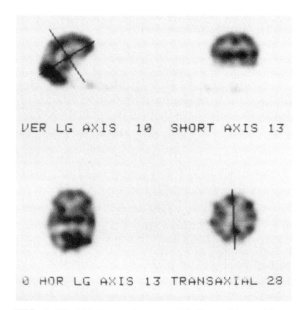

VER LG AXIS   10   SHORT AXIS 13

0 HOR LG AXIS 13 TRANSAXIAL 28

FIG. 8–13. (A) Rotated transaxial slice, with positional plane marked for perpendicular reorientation. **(B)** Sagittal view with positional plane identified for horizontal, and, thus, true transaxial reorientation. **(C)** Final transaxial view after correction for poor patient positioning during acquisition.

draws a stright line through the right and left hemispheres at the angle of the tilt (Fig. 8–13A). This will generate a series of sagittal slices that are void of the patient's acquired angle. The user then is prompted to place a line that will be indicative of coronal slice generation (Fig. 8–13B). This is the point at which the user may compensate for the hyperextension of the mandible and produce a series of realistic coronal and transaxial slice (Fig. 8–13C).

The physician diagnosing the brain study also should be cognizant of the rotational variabilities that are possible with SPECT. If, for example, a patient were referred for a perfusion brain study to explain an aphasia that might be temporal lobe related, the first reaction of the image interpreter would be to look for an asymmetry of the temporal horns in a number of the lower cut transaxial slices (Fig. 8–14). Both the technologist and physician should be aware, however, that a patient who is positioned for acquisition with the head cocked to one side may produce transaxial slices that stimulate temporal lobe asymmetry. This conflict may be avoided

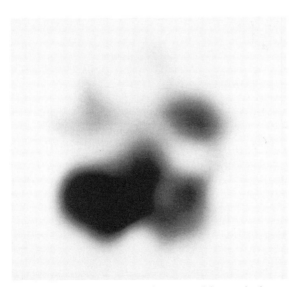

FIG. 8–14. Asymmetry of temporal horns in lower transaxial slice of patient with aphasia. Care must be taken to ensure proper patient positioning during acquisition before making a diagnosis from this transaxial slice.

if the complete data set, including the raw projections, are reviewed for positional discrepancies.

Single Slice Limitations

As previously mentioned numerous times, reliance on single slices for a diagnosis may be equated to reading a whole-body bone scan from only one static view of the lumbar spine. There is a great deal of information in all the transaxial, coronal, and sagittal slices. A number of software programs are commercially available that attempt and are often sucessful at portraying the complete set of transaxial slices as total-organ three-dimensional images. Figure 8–15A presents a transaxial, coronal, and sagittal slice of an ^{123}I-amine brain study. A defect is well demonstrated in the right frontal lobe and, based on the patient's history, probably indicative of a stroke. The set of transaxial slices are reprocessed with a three-dimensional reprojection technique, and the application of a gradient shade program, to produce a set of images that truly look like a brain. The complete extent of the stroke is clearly demonstrated with this technique in comparison to the single slice images (Fig. 8–15B).

SUMMARY

The idea that the transition from planar imaging to SPECT is not technically overwhelming has been portrayed throughout this book. There are, however, exceptions, and with SPECT, in particular, the exception is brain perfusion studies. Whether the radiopharmaceutical employed is labeled to ^{123}I or ^{99m}Tc, all the variables that may possibly degrade a brain SPECT study seem to be amplified. The reduction of resolution and contrast due to the detector target distant and imposed by the patient's shoulders is a constant source of limited quality image production. More importantly, the compressed information density, resulting from the bulk of primary photons arising from a relatively small homogenous area as compared to the detector's field of view, is subject to seemingly amplified artifact generation as a function of inadequate quality control. The issue is complicated further by the fact that a number

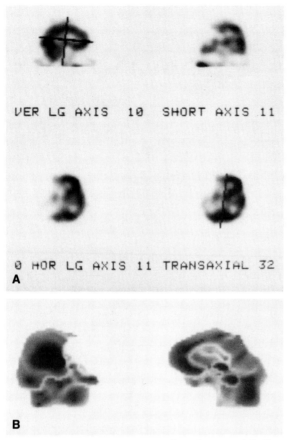

VER LG AXIS   10   SHORT AXIS 11

0 HOR LG AXIS 11 TRANSAXIAL 32

A

B

FIG. 8–15. (A) Sagittal, coronal, and transaxial slices of an ^{123}I-IMP brain study presenting with a left middle cerebral artery stroke. **(B)** Distance-weighted reprojection of the same study demonstrating the complete extent of affected area.

of patients who require this study are not always responsive to lengthy attempts at immobility, making SPECT brain perfusion studies a truly demanding technical challenge. The process, however, is not impossible. A review of 400 perfusion brain studies, performed by one of the authors, using ^{123}I iodoamphetamine revealed only four that were technically undiagnostic, and two that could not be, due to lack of patient cooperation, acquired at all. Patient cooperation in this study varied from hostile to placid. With

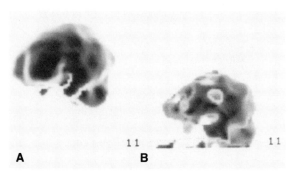

A   **B**

FIG. 8–16. (A) Distant-weighted reprojection in the
LAO 30° projection of a normal 32-yr-old male and
(B) a 29-yr-old i.v. drug abuser.

some patience and experience, however, any technologist with any
SPECT unit should be able to institute a reliable perfusion brain
SPECT protocol. Table 8–2 offers recommendations that may be
useful.

Table 8-2. Protocol for SPECT Brain Perfusion Studies

Acquisition

1. Agent and dose:	3–5mCi, ^{123}I-iodoamphetamine
2. Collimators:	LEAP (bore length = 40-mm) Medium-energy (bore length = 25-mm)
3. Computer:	360°, 64 × 64 matrix 64 projections, 35 sec/projections
4. Time of study:	40 min

Processing

1. Uniformity correction:	Extrinsic with ^{123}I
2. Pre-filter:	Hann with 0.5 rolloff or Butterworth with 0.25 cutoff per 20 power
3. Reconstruction:	Ramp filter (999 cutoff)
4. Attenuation correction:	Yes, μ = 0.40

Display

1. Sagittal/Coronal:	Yes, 1-slice thick if positioning correct
2. Oblique reconstruction:	Yes, if patient position is incorrect

SUGGESTED READINGS

1. Holman BL, Hill TC, Magistretti PL. Brain imaging with emission computed tomography and radiolabeled amines. *Invest Radiol* 1982; 17:206–215.

2. Neirinckx RD, Canning LR, Piper IM, et al. Technetium-99m-d, 1-HM-PAO: A new radiopharmaceutical for SPECT imaging of regional cerebral blood perfusion. *J Nucl Med* 1987;28:191–202.

3. Royal HD, Hill TC, Holman BL. Clinical brain imaging with isopropyl-iodoamphetamine and SPECT. *Semin Nucl Med* 1985;15:357–375.

4. Holman BL, Hill TC, Polak JF, et al. Cerebral perfusion imaging with iodine-123-labeled amines. *Arch Neurol* 1984;41:1060–1063.

5. Polak JF, Holman BL, Moretti JL, et al. I-123 HIPDM brain imaging with a rotating gamma camera and slant-hole collimator. *J Nucl Med* 1984;25:495–498.

6. Polak JF, English RJ, Holman BL. Performance of collimators used for tomographic imaging of I-123 contaminated with I-124. *J Nucl Med* 1983;24:1065–1069.

7. Tsui BMW, Gullberg GT, Edgerton ER, et al. Design and clinical utility of a fan beam collimator for SPECT imaging of the head. *J Nucl Med* 1986;27:810–819.

8. Cohen MB, Graham LS, Lake R, et al. Diagnosis of Alzheimer's disease and multiple infarct dementia by tomographic imaging of iodine-123 IMP. *J Nucl Med* 1986;27:769–774.

9. English RJ, Holman BL. Current status of cerebral perfusion radiopharmaceuticals. *J Nucl Technol* 1987;15:30–35.

9 MYOCARDIAL PERFUSION SPECT

The single most common reason for purchasing a single-photon emission computed tomography (SPECT) system, whether at a university hospital or a walk-in clinic, appears to be for imaging myocardial perfusion with thallium-201 (^{201}Tl). Long considered less than the ideal radionuclide, ^{201}Tl presents a host of problems and technical considerations that, at times, make quality planar imaging an art. The energy level of the radionuclide, the anatomy and orientation of the heart, and the size of the organ present a set of conditions that are not unlike those encountered in brain perfusion SPECT, described in Chapter 8. The only real difference, however, is that the nuclear medicine community is use to, and for the most part, comfortable with ^{201}Tl planar imaging, thus allowing SPECT to enter as an unintrusive improvement.

Scintigraphic technology has become an increasingly important noninvasive method of assessing myocardial perfusion. Radionuclides that have been employed for this purpose include radioisotopes of potassium, rubidium, and, of course, thallium. It is only because ^{201}Tl has physical characteristics less complicated than potassium and rubidium, that is has been able to remain the choice for myocardial perfusion scintigraphy.

The clinical application of myocardial scintigraphy has been limited by these physical and physiological characteristics, leading many researchers to seek alternative technetium-99m compounds. Thallium's relatively long half-life (72 hr) restricts the injected dose

to 2 to 3 mCi, presenting difficult length of acquisition time deci-
sions, and making serial evaluation of myocardial perfusion difficult. Its low-energy mercury x-ray peak (69–83 keV) is not ideally
suited for clinical gamma cameras; photon attenuation causes inaccuracies in quantitation and three-dimensional reconstructions.
In addition, because myocardial distribution of ^{201}Tl is rapid, it
reflects flow for a relatively short period of time after stress. Furthermore, when injected at rest, its myocardial uptake relative to
background activity is often poor, and finally, since it is cyclotron
produced, it has availability limitations and possible cost burdens.

At this point, the new user to SPECT is probably asking; Why
bother? The cards are all stacked against me? Simply put, placing aside all the debate concerning acquisition techniques,
redistribution concerns, processing methods, etc., SPECT removes
over- and underlying tissue and background interference, presents
a complete view of the left ventrical, and is relatively easy to perform. The authors emphasize this last point with a comment.
Thallium-201 SPECT is not difficult, if the user understands and
accepts that whatever method of acquisition and processing they
should employ will be subject to criticism from users who do it
some other way. If users should decide to collect thallium data in
a 180-degree arc, then they are at odds with the 360-degree fac-
tion. If static images are collected prior to tomographic acquisition, then the rapid redistribution advocates will find fault.
Whichever course a user chooses to follow or preach does not
diminish the fact that the routine collection and processing of [201]Tl
data is not technically, or logistically, complicated. With the pros
and cons stated, the user may proceed to establish a ^{201}Tl protocol
(see Table 9–1) keeping the following six points in mind; (1) quality control, (2) patient positioning, (3) acquisition, (4) reconstruction filters and windows, (5) image reorientation and display, and
(6) quantitation techniques.

QUALITY CONTROL

As has been stated before, proper integrity of the SPECT system
must be established before patient acquisition begins. There may
be a tendency to ignore high statistic uniformity correction and

Table 9-1. Protocol for Myocardial Perfusion SPECT

Acquisition

1. Agent and dose:	2–3mCi, ^{120}Tl
2. Collimator:	LEAP
3. Computer:	180°, 64 × 64 matrix 64 projections, 20–25 sec/projections
4. Time of study:	27–30 min

Processing

1. Uniformity correction:	Extrinsic 30 million counts
2. Pre-filter:	Hann with 04 to 05 0.5 rolloff
3. Reconstruction:	Ramp filter (999 cutoff)
4. Attenuation correction:	No

Display

1. Long and short axis reorientation, 1 slice thick
2. Repeat with same methodology for rest study

center of rotation requirements once a user has become comfortable with thallium tomography. This is probably because it appears very difficult to produce poor cross-sectional images. It will appear to the new user that the left ventrical is presented as a doughnut whether uniformity corrected or not. This is an unreliable approach, especially if some method of quantitation is to be employed, because nonvisual count variances may be significantly altered from a systems nonconformities.

This philosophy also remains true with center of rotation (COR) correction. Improper COR factors will result in a smearing of counts across the image matrix. As was demonstrated with the point source in Chapter 7, a point of activity may be reconstructed as a doughnut. Therefore, it stands to reason that an object that should be viewed as a doughnut, such as a mid-slice of the left ventricle, might well take on some whole new geometric design, should the COR be substantially off the mark. The real problem is that these artifacts may not be as obvious as those that might be seen with tomography of some other organ such as the brain or liver. The user who does not verify the COR, or apply uniformity correction may produce a visually acceptable left ventricle, but the distribution of counts and any subsequent quantification attempts may lack the integrity of a well-controlled examination.

PATIENT POSITIONING

The two most common mistakes that appear as a result of incorrect positioning result from (a) patient's discomfort, and (b) misplacement of the heart on the projection matrix in some projections. The first is an understandable condition, and not always within the power of the technologist to correct. The patient is required to raise his/her left arm above the head and out of the field of view for a 180-degree acquisition, and both arms for a 360-degree collection. This can be a tiresome exercise to perform for 20 to 30 min, especially if the patient has some form of shoulder problem, such as bursitis. In any case, motion of the heart is subject to any up and down movement of the left arm. The result would, of course, be a degradation of slice-to-slice resolution. Therefore, it should be explained to the patient that once the arm is up, it must stay there.

The most comfortable position for a patient seems to be one in which the left forearm is placed along the forehead and given some type of strap to grip. This may be easily done by wrapping a loose length of tape around the head of the table, prior to the patients appearance, and under the pillow, forming a long loop. Once the patient is positioned on the table, with his/her arm resting on the forehead, the loop may be placed in his/her left hand as a support mechanism, similar to the strap found on subway trains or streetcars. Again, the technologist should make sure that the patient has no rolled up sheets or matress digging into the shoulders or back, causing even a small degree of discomfort. One should try to keep in mind that even a minimally slight degree of pressure in the back will intensify as a function of time, even for as short a period as 20 min. After all, even an amount of time as small as 1 sec becomes lengthy when ones hand is on a hot stove.

The second instance of mispositioning concerns proper placement of the target on the collection matrix from all projections. The left ventricle is subject to falling out of the field of view because of its anatomic location. As a rule, the left ventricle is anterior and to the left of the sternum. If a 180-degree acquisition is employed, acquisition might begin in the right anterior oblique (RAO) 30-degree position, and finalize in the left posterior oblique (LPO) 30-degree projection. With these extremes, the left ventricle may slide very close to the edge of the collection matrix of the detectors field of view, and in some cases completely out of the field of view. This is usually true if the target is not positioned in the true center of the rotational field of view from both an anterior position and a left lateral position. One must keep in mind that most scintillation detectors are circular, with the largest field of view at the center or the detector's longest diameter. For example, a detector with a 41-cm diameter will demonstrate decreasing diameter widths in the directions of both the patient's head and feet. Therefore, should the left ventricle be positioned in the lower or upper one-third of the camera from the anterior or LAO 30-degree view, it will in all probability be missing in the initial projections collected at the beginning of the study, as well as those final frames toward the end of acquisition. When the patient is positioned, and the computer's parameters established, the technologist should engage the persist scope or position mode and monitor the left ventricle in the RAO 30-degree, anterior, LAO 45-degree, and LPO 30-degree positions verifying that the target is always in the center of the greatest portion of the detectors diameter, and thus always within the field of view. This, of course, is not quite as critical with rectangular head detectors, for the field of view width never decreases.

ACQUISITION PARAMETERS

Before any collection parameters may be discussed, one fundamental decision must be made that is unique to thallium myocardial SPECT. Will the data be collected in a 180-degree arc, or a complete 360-degree circle? As mentioned in Chapter 4 and at the beginning of this chapter, literature supporting both techniques are plentiful, and arguments for and against both are valid. A quick review of these pros and cons might be warranted to assist the new user in making this first protocol decision.

Generally speaking, proponents of the 180-degree collection method point to data that states the majority of counts and usable data originate from the left anterior side of the chest, and that those photons that might be detected from the right posterior portions of the chest are compromised by spine and lung/rib attenuation. The 180-degree advocates justify the inability to properly, mathematically correct for attenuation, and to the philosophy that no attenuation correction is better than falsely attempting to correct for an organ surrounded by so many tissue types with as many varying attenuation coefficients. If one is employing an attenuation correction algorithm that institutes a single correction coefficient (mu), then which should be used, the coefficient for bone, air, soft tissue, or fluid? All of these photon attenuating masses may be found surrounding the left ventricle of the heart.

One the other hand, 360-degree advocates state that the 180-degree technique is primarily a tool for reduced acquisition time. They also state that the 180-degree arc yields distortion, and produces artifact generation similar to that produced by other limited angle techniques, namely the seven pinhole collimator method. This segment of the nuclear medicine community points to studies indicating that insufficient and inconsistent count collections will yield inaccurate distributions in the reconstructed image. For example, posterior portions of the left ventricle may not be truly reflected in the reconstruction slices because insufficient counts were collected from that region. This certainly has a ring of practicality to it, for most 180-degree collection methods stop collecting in the LPO position. Should the posterior/inferior walls of the left ventricle be count deficient, the user is left with the problem of deciding whether this abnormality is the physiologic truth, or the result of a technologic camouflage.

At this juncture, the new user is most probably still confused about which technique to employ, and would simply appreciate a straightforward direction with which to start. It appears at present, that the mainstream nuclear medicine community is sticking with the 180-degree acquisition technique, and those users looking for a minimally controversial place to start might follow this path. It is important, however, that the new user not utilize this collection method with thoughts of reduced acquisition times in mind. This has often been proposed as a plus for the 180-degree method and is completely misleading. As with any scintigraphic exam, quality image production is dependent on adequate statistics. The user who considers collecting 64 projections in 360°, at 30 sec per projection, cannot simply collect 32 projections in 180° for the same time per projection and expect the same statistical quality. The information density will have been reduced by one-half with this philosophy, increasing noise and artifact. Also, one must keep in mind that the angular sampling of this method has been reduced by one-half, substantially decreasing the effectiveness of the reconstruction filter function (Ramp filter), again generating more artifact.

As mentioned in Chapter 4, adequate angular sampling for clincal studies falls within parameters that, on the low end of the scale, yield artifact-generating images, to the extreme end that eats up disk space and computer time while offering no practical visual improvement in clinical image quality. In practical terms, if three choices of projection numbers per 180-degree acquisition are offered; 32, 64, and 128, the most reasonable choice would be 64. Of course the total time of patient acquisition remains basically would be reduced by one-half with each doubling of calibrated projections. Again, the time of processing and need for disk space appear not to justify the use of 128 projections at 10 sec per projection, because of the noise and statistical inaccuracies inherent in clinical data.

Summerizing the above statements, a conservative, mainstream approach to thallium tomographic acquisition might start with 64 projections collected in a 180-degree arc, for 24 sec per projection, with a 2–3 mCi administered dose of the radiopharmaceutical during peak exercise testing. There are two more details related to acquisition that deserve attention, however; with what view should data collection begin, and what matrix size one should consider.

The question of thallium redistribution was mentioned earlier, and to some degree has a bearing on what position the beginning of data collection should start. There have been reports in the literature that redistribution of ^{201}Tl may begin as early as 17 min following exercise testing, posing something of a dilemma for an acquisition process that takes 25 min. For example, should a SPECT collection process take 25 min to complete, and the study's initial projection be the RAO 30-degree view, is it conceivable that redistribution takes place in the posterior portions of the left ventricle by the time the detector reaches the left lateral throught LPO projections? If this is the case, would it not be advisable to begin acquisition in the LPO 30-degree projection, and collect counterclockwise until the RAO 30-degree view is reached? This could, however, compromise the detected distribution of the septal wall, acquired best from the anterior through RAO projections. One can appreciate the conflicts, and quite frankly, there is no magic answer should rapid redistribution take place as reported in some of the literature.

One approach might be to begin acquisition in that projection that best meets the clinical situation. For example, if the patient is referred for thallium exercise testing to determine the degree of ischemia possibly present in the posterior or lateral wall, then the start of tomographic acquisition might best begin in the LPO 30-degree projection, and continue counterclockwise. This approach would seem, however, to be somewhat impractical as very few referrals show up in a nuclear medicine department with a requisition, never mind a detailed history. Thus, the truly conservative approach to this problem is to collect two or three static images immediately after exercise testing, and employ the tomographic slices as an enhancement tool. This method might be of paricular value to the new user, for the security of a known technique is not lost and a little insurance for a new technology is provided. As a degree of familiarity and confidence in the SPECT interpretation is gained, dropping one or perhaps even all the static views might be considered.

Selection of a matrix size is not nearly as complicated as some of the other acquisition choices that have been described. The majority of commercial systems provide the user with two basic choices, a 64×64 matrix, or a 128×128 matrix. At first glance, the higher resolution of the 128×128 matrix would seem to be the correct choice to make. But again, as with other organs described, the minimal gain in resolution is offset by the reduction in information density, and the requirements for increased processing time and contiguous disk space. The use of a zoom mode of 1.5 with a 64×64 matrix, has been suggested as one way of limiting disk space requirements while increasing the matrix size and resultant image resolution. While this technqiue has proven somewhat effective in perfusion brain SPECT, it is positionally difficult with the heart. As mentioned before in patient positioning, the left ventricle is anterior and in the left chest. In 180-degree acquisition, the myocardium tends to sweep from the right side of the field in the RAO projections to the left side of the field of view in the LAO projections, often coming very close to the edge of the detectors field of view, even with a 1.0 zoom. Increasing or employing an increased zoom mode reduces the detectors usable field of view, substantially raising the probability of the left ventricle falling out of the collection matrix from any number of projections. Any negligable gain in resolution would effectively be negated with the loss of data, and increased artifact generation caused by the hearts removal from any number of acquisition frames. Therfore, the safest and least complicated technique is to collect thallium studies onto a 64 × 64 matrix with a standard 1.0 zoom mode.

One final note on establishing acquisition parameters for SPECT that also applies to standard static imaging. The vast majority of today's gamma cameras employ triple peaking capabilities. There are a number of usable photons that originate from ^{201}Tl in the 135- and 160-keV range that are often ignored. The technologist seeking a modest increase in counts per unit should give consideration to initiating dual or triple peaking that would include the gamma photons from these regions.

RECONSTRUCTION

The low count collection of thallium tomography appears to provide very little innovative selection of filter/window combinations. Liver studies, for instance, may yield substantial numbers of counts per projection and reduced statistical noise influence, allowing the user any number of filter options while attempting to extract high quality data. Due to limited dose administration and less than optimal target to background ratios, selection of filter/window reconstruction parameters for thallium tomographic data seems restricted to the degree of "smoothing" with which an intepreting physician becomes accustom.

The many filters presented throughout this text may be inappropriately broken down into two basic categories—the high band-pass (Butterworth, Metz, etc.), and the low bandpass (Hamming, Hann, Parzen, etc.). The high bandpass filters may be very effective in extrapolating data, and reducing noise, but require a great deal of study before implementation. Reconstructed data that exists in the higher frequencies is most often noise, and when included in reconstruction, produces a bumping, or more properly termed, ringing effect. The high bandpass filters employ a power function that alters the amplitude, or height of data to be reconstructed, and if not applied correctly, may well amplify the noise that is included, resulting in excessive ringing. Again, this noise exists at the far end of the x axis, and a high power factor applied with a high rolloff will cause reconstruction of artificially high noise. And, of course, thallium studies are loaded with noise.

Therefore, the safest way to get started with thallium reconstruction is to employ a low bandpass filter such as the Hamming or Hann. These filters have no power function, and tend to be symmetrical with a mild rolloff, allowing for a greater margin of error in where the cutoff may take place. Because there is less incidence of ringing with these filters, the basic result is one of visual smoothing. If the 64 × 64 matrix is used for collection, a Hann window with a 0.5 cutoff will produce a moderate degree of smoothing while retaining some sharpness. Moving the cutoff to 0.8 or 0.9 will result in an excessive graininess, while reducing the cutoff to 0.25 or 0.3 will virtually smooth out any concept of detail and resolution. The difference between the Hamming, Hann, and Parzen is basically the slope of the rolloff and the degree of the amplitude. The Hamming filter appears to be the best for accepting usable data, while the Parzen tends to supress much of what might be desired. The Hann is a middle of the road approach.

There are a number of alternative methods to invoking a window function with the Ramp filter that may or may not be optimal. Consider for a moment that the data to be filtered exist in three direction, the x direction representing side to side of the transaxial slice, the y direction going from top to bottom, and the z direction parallel to the axis of rotation, or the data represented from the first slice through the last. Ideally, one would hope that a filter function would take into account the relationship between pixels in all three directions. However, if a window is applied to the Ramp filter after the reconstruction process, then the image is actually smoothed, or filtered, in only the two-dimensional place of the individual transaxial slice. There is no filtered relationship between neighboring slices. This may be corrected by one of two ways, prefiltering the raw projection set prior to reconstruction, or applying a "y" filter to each transaxial slice following reconstruction. This last technique may not be available on all commercially available systems, and has been described in Chapter 5.

Prefiltering the projection set allows the user a bit of flexability, while establishing a filter relationship in the z direction. Prefiltering is actually not unlike temporal smoothing of a dynamic or gated data set, in that each frame is related to its ajoining neighbor. Thus, if a Hann, or Hamming filter with a 0.5 rolloff is applied to the projection set prior to reconstruction, and the filter projection set reconstructed with a Ramp filter, a transaxial set of slices will be produced that show a relationship in all three directions.

One final note on the reconstruction process. The use of attenuation correction, as previously metioned, appears to be an unrealistic effort. In 180-degree acquisition, there are no opposing projections that would be required to employ some effective attenuation correction algorithm, and if 360-degree collection were used, the decision on what attenuation coefficient to be employed would seem at best to be a flip of the coin. Therfore, ignoring the effects of attenuation when doing thallium SPECT doesn't seem like a radical concept. Keep in mind, if quantification of stress and rest thallium tomography is to be attempted, the effects of attenuation would be the same for both studies and would cancel each other out in any ratio calculations.

IMAGE REORIENTATION AND DISPLAY

As mentioned in Chapter 5, the heart does not sit in any convenient acquisition or reconstruction plane. The left ventricle usually exist with the base to apex axis lying from 15 ° to 45 ° from the z axis of the table, producing transaxial images that are often an anatomic mystery to the new user. Thus the need for some reorien-

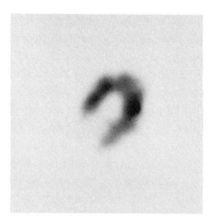

FIG. 9-1. Mid-ventricular trans-axial slice presenting a typical horse-shoe appearance that provides little anatomic relationships. For example, is the lack of perfusion in the posterior region a defect, or normal appearance of the valve plane?

tation method is a must. Software for this purpose exists on every system and requires little practice to implement.

Figure 9-1 demonstrates a mid-ventricle transaxial slice with two opposing walls angled ~ 15° to the readers right. The patients anterior aspect is at the top of the page and the posterior at the bottom. The core of the problem exists with determining where the apex and base exist as complete, independent entities. In this particular slice the approximate 30-degree angle from the sternum, of the apex to base plane, places a small amount of both regions on the same transaxial slice. The user is then left with the problem, for example, of determining which region of the posterior portion of the left ventricle is reduced-thallium uptake a result of disease, or the valve plane that naturally exists at the base . On many occasions, the cold region at the posterior portion of the heart will occupy the whole transaxial slice set. Simply put, the normal left ventricle should not consist of a valve plane that is so large it occupies all slices; however, the angle of the apex to base plane is often such, in the normal patient, that the horseshoe appearance of the ventricle is evident in virtually all these slices.

Thus, it becomes necessary to straighten this whole set of trans-axial images into a group of planes that have distinctive planes related to anatomic landmarks of the left ventricle, and not the body as a whole. This may be accomplished by rearranging the cube, or volume of pixels containing the stack of transaxial slices in such a way that three new sets of slices are generated.

Each manufacturer produces software that may vary slightly from its competitors, though the basic principles remain the same. Figure 9–2 demonstrates the first step in this reorientation process carried out on one typical commercial system. The transaxial image is presented to the user as a starting point for producing new planes, and asks that the user place a line between and parallel to two opposing walls (Fig. 9–3). This action will, in effect, turn the stack of transaxial slices to a stright 0-180-degree verticle plane, and begin to generate a series of slices at a 90-degree angle to this plane (Fig. 9–4). These slices are, in effect, sagittal slices of an apex to base orientation. The user is then instructed to identify the apex, base, anterior, and posterior walls, and place another line parallel to these two walls (Fig. 9–5). Completion of this process will then generate anterior-to-posterior slices (something of a coronal nature), and apex-to-base slices, sometimes called cucumber slices. The complete effort will result in three sets of slices generated from the original transaxial set, and at 90-degree angles to the apex-to-base plane (Fig. 9–6).

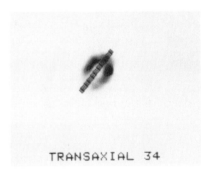

TRANSAXIAL 34

FIG. 9–2. Reorientation of the left ventrical into long- and short-axis slices first requires the user to identify the angle of paralleled walls from a mid-ventricular transaxial slice.

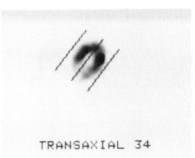

TRANSAXIAL 34

FIG. 9–3. Placement of cursors between the parallel walls will, in effect, rotate the transaxial set counterclockwise in preparation for lateral slice generation.

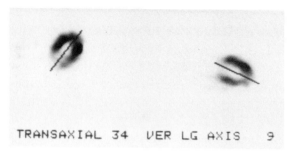

FIG. 9–4. Vertical long-axis (sagittal) slices are displayed allowing the user to identify the angle vetween the apex and the base.

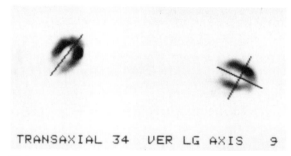

FIG. 9–5. Generation of horizontal long-axis (coronal) and short-axis (cucumber) slices begin from the user defined angles placed in the sagittal reference set.

This process is, of course, repeated for the rest views in what should be the same manner as was the stress study. It is important that the parallel reference lines used for the stress study be applied to the rest, so that reproducable methodology be employed. With both the exercise and rest study reconstructed and reorientated, the data should be presented in some systematic manner that allows the intepreting physician to easily compare the two studies. Display techniques are a matter of individual tastes varying from institution to institution, and from software package to software package.

Software is one exciting aspect of SPECT that appears to have unlimited boundries. While the basic process of reconstruction and reorientation is an accomplishment in its own right, researchers and manufacturers are developing even more advanced programs

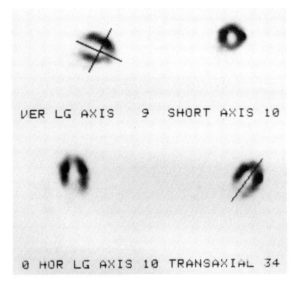

FIG. 9-6. The completed reorientation process presents the user with three angles of slice generation that account for variances in the left ventricals normal anatomic placement.

that present cross sections in rotating, three-dimensional movies. Figure 9–7 presents one view of thallium distribution in the left ventricle of the heart during peak exercise and again at rest. This particular view is one of 64, encompassing a 360-degree rotation, while Figure 9–8 demonstrates other viewing angles. When placed in a cine mode, both studies spin about a superior-inferior axis giving a visual impression of a rotating left ventricle. The images which are produced display three-dimensional isocount level surfaces, shaded so that brightness decreases linearly with the distance of the surface from the viewing plane. The visual impressions, while yet to be clinically validated, are of a truly dramatic nature.

QUANTITATION TECHNIQUES

A great deal of effort has been expended in the search for reliable quantitative measurements of thallium distribution in the heart. The most basic technique is to simply place regions of interest throughout the left ventricle, extrapolate the counts, and compare

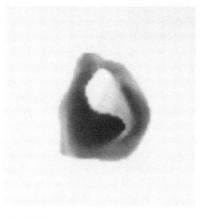

FIG. 9–7. Three-dimensional surface mapping of a left ventrical, looking anteriorly from the apex to base, demonstrating an anterior/septal perfusion defect at exercise.

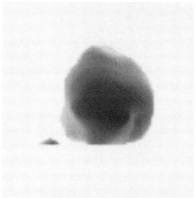

FIG. 9–8. The same three-dimensional surface map of the left ventrical at the rest phase.

between exercise and rest. The drawback to this technique, is of course, user-to-user variability, the number of ROIs and tomographic slices, and, of course, the time of analysis. Other software techniques are becoming available that attempt to limit the number of outside variables, reduce the time of processing, and present the complete transxial or oblique set as one composite, quantifiable image.

One technique of standardizing quantitation is the circumferential profile. This process examines a selected slice, usually a "cucumber slice", by placing a circular region of interest around the exterior and interior complete wall of the left ventricles "doughnut-shaped" slice, and plotting the counts on a standard x, y coordinate system as a function of radial distance. For example, the anterior/septal wall may be designated the starting point of the *x* axis, and the counts plotted as some function of distance around a clockwise pattern. The process may be repeated for the rest studies, and both curves corrected for decay and washout. The exercise curve may then be subtracted from the rest, and a resultant curve presented that reflects redistribution of thallium.

An alternative quanitative process for thallium SPECT is the "Bulls-eye program". An understanding of this technique requires the reader to visualize a stacking of the short-axis (cucumber) slices, and view the stack from the apex onto the base, with each slice artificially spreading out in a circular pattern as a function of its distance from the apex (Fig. 9–9). With each wall identified, a sembance of coronary anatomy could be mapped, and exercise/stress relationships deduced.

The quantitative methods described are relative in nature and don't address the concepts of volume measurement, for good reason. The problems of attenuation and scatter correction, combined with partial volume effects make absolute quantitation and volume calculations extremely difficult. Partial volume effects, for example, are inherent factors that should be considered in all interpretations of tomographic data, whether visual or quantitative. For example, a central slice of the left ventricle contains portions of both its neighboring slices. It becomes difficult to attempt a volume determination of that slice without first establishing the impact of its adjoining slices.

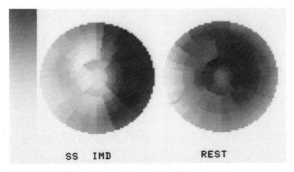

SS IMD   REST

FIG. 9–9. Exercise and rest "bull's-eye" plot presenting mild redistribution of the septal wall.

SUMMARY

Myocardial perfusion SPECT with ^{201}Tl is becoming a well-established technique in the nuclear medicine community. While the radiopharmaceutical itself has a number of suboptimal characteristics, the technology and instrumentation of today's rotating gamma cameras yield images of relatively high quality. The addition of the ^{99m}Tc myocardial perfusion agents will, of course, produce even higher quality tomographic scintigraphs, possibly in shorter periods of acquisition times. For the new user of thallium SPECT, the following recommendations are presented as a starting point.

SUGGESTED READINGS

1. Maublant J, Cassagnes J, LeJeune JJ, et al. A comparison between conventional scintigraphy and emission tomography with thallium-201 in the detection of myocardial infarction: Concise communication. *J Nucl Med* 1982;23:204–208.

2. Prigent FM, Maddahi J, Garcia E, et al. Thallium-201 stress-redistribution myocardial rotational tomography: Development of criteria for visual interpretation. *Am Heart J* 1985;109:274–281.

3. Garcia EV, Van Train K, Maddahi J, et al. Quantification of rotational thallium-201 myocardial tomography. *J Nucl Med* 1985;26:17–26.

4. Eisner R, Churchwell A, Noever T, et al. Quantitative analysis of the tomographic thallium-201 myocardial bull's eye display: Critical role of correcting for patient motion. *J Nucl Med* 1988;29:91–97.

5. Geckle WJ, Frank TL, Links JM, et al. Correction for patient and organ movement in SPECT: Application to exercise thallium-201 cardiac imaging. *J Nucl Med* 1988;29:441–450.

6. Friedman J, Van Train K, Maddahi J, et al. "Upward creep" of the heart: A frequent source of false-positive reversible defects during thallium-201 stress-redistribution SPECT. *J Nucl Med* 1989;30:1718–1722.

7. Gutman J, Berman DS, Freeman M, et al. Time to completed redistribution of thallium-201 in exercise myocardial scintigraphy: Relationship to the degree of coronary stenosis. *Am Heart J* 1983;106:989–995.

10 LIVER, BONE AND GALLIUM SPECT

Chapters 8 and 9 dealt with the establishment of brain and myocardial perfusion SPECT on an individual basis, because of specialized applications and problems. While brain perfusion SPECT may appear to be an examination of the future, and thallium SPECT a function of a nuclear medicine units cardiac volume, the day-to-day applications of SPECT in routine clinical studies still remains an underappreciated tool.

The initiation of SPECT into the daily scintigraphic grind is one of surprising technical ease. The problem that does present itself the most often is not one of technical quality, but one of logistics. The clinical unit with one or two rotating gamma cameras more often than not shies away from SPECT because of unwarranted fears of extensive camera time, and possibly reduced, or backed up, throughput. At most, SPECT should never add more than an average of 30 min to an examination time, and proper advanced planning will not diminish the volume output of any nuclear medicine department.

Throughout this text, a great deal of emphasis has been placed on the need for adequate study information density, proper quality control, and careful patient positioning. And, while these and many more factors play an important role in the production of diagnostic tomographic images, the most important variable in the process is the patient. The statement that SPECT should add no more than 30 min to a given study is not based on some physical or biologic question, but on the common sense approach to basic patient care.

Put in perspective, it is clear that the average healthy individual begins to get uncomfortable and restless after one-half hour in the same position, increasing the probability of movement with each additional minute. Thus, it would be somewhat unrealistic that a technologist or physician should expect the ill, or seriously ill patient to remain motionless for greater periods of time in order to gain more statistics. Keep in mind that should proper collection parameters be dictated by a formula that states that 1-hr acquisition time is mandatory and the patient rolls over on one side in the middle of the exam, the end result is reconstructed garbage. Therefore, the time of the study's acquisition is not so much dependent on some textbook formula as it is on a technologist's estimate of a patient's mental and physical tolerance for remaining immobile.

LIVER SPECT

Liver SPECT with ^{99m}Tc-sulfur colloid or labeled red blood cells (RBCs) is perhaps the easiest technically, and least time-consuming of all the SPECT studies. The liver is large and usually homogeneous, has a high target-to-background ratio, does not redistribute or washout sulfur colloid, and usually yields high count rates. A search through the literature reveals a number of papers that claim a higher sensitivity, specificity, and accuracy for sulfur colloid liver SPECT than for conventional scintigraphic liver imaging. The reason that liver SPECT is not as popular as it might be, is not so much a result of the technology or time involved, as it is the decline in liver scintigraphy, in general, because of the high resolution of CT and MRI. Because liver studies are not as overwhelming in day-to-day scheduling as they might once have been, incorporating the SPECT component into the routine liver protocol is not something that will considerably disrupt a day's schedule.

Quality Control

The liver is particularly susceptible to poorly corrected uniformity variations. It is large, homogenous, and generally without back-

formation densities. A sulfur colloid study may have 200,000 counts per projection, but the counts may be located in half the number of pixels, requiring a higher filter cutoff. A RBC liver study may also have 200,000 counts per projection, however, spread out over all 4,096 pixels of a 64 × 64 matrix, requiring a lower rolloff value. Second, the type of defect being sought may influence a filter/window selection. The sulfur colloid study usually searches for "cold" defects, a much more difficult task than searching for the "hot" spots, characteristic of a hemangioma in a RBC study. Thus, the use of excessive smoothing may have greater consequences with the sulfur colloid study than with the RBC study.

As with thallium and brain studies, the use of prefiltering the liver projection set is also recommended. Prefiltering with the filter and rolloff of choice provides a temporal effect between projection frames that translates into a semblance of continuity between transaxial slice, or a type of smoothing effect in the z direction of the transaxial slice set.

The phantom studies presented in Chapter 7 and 8 are applicable to liver SPECT for demonstrating the alterations of reconstructed counts with the application of decreasing rolloff values. If the user is aware of what lower limit may be employed, before data is sererely affected, then the choice of a filter/window combination becomes one of individual taste. Figure 10–2 presents a series of liver (^{99m}Tc-RBCs) transaxial slices collected on a 64 × 64 matrix reconstructed with a Ramp/Hann filter and varying rolloffs, providing the user with an overview of filtering effects.

Also included as part of the reconstruction process is the need for attenuation correction. Because the liver occupies such a large portion of the reconstruction matrix, attenuation correction becomes an absolute necessity. Unlike thallium SPECT, however, the liver presents an excellent set of conditions for attenuation correction. As a target, it is generally uniform, homogenous, and composed of one attenuation mass, requiring only one calculated attenuation coefficient. This is not to say that the attenuation correction techniques available are perfect, they are just better than nothing. Figure 10–3A presents a RBC liver study that was reconstructed without any correction for attenuation, resulting in an image with noticable edge activity. Figure 10–3B demonstrates the

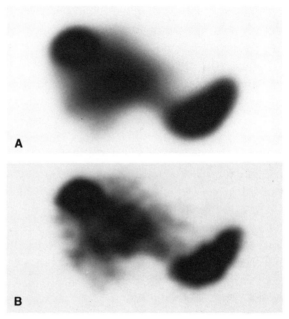

FIG. 10-2. (265K count/projection) Transaxial slice of a ⁹⁹ᵐTc-labeled RBC liver study reconstructed with a Ramp filter and Hann window at rolloffs of (**A**) 0.25 and (**B**) 0.50.

same slice after the introduction of an attenuation correction factor, and the resultant uniform appearance of the count distribution.

BONE SPECT

As an extension of standard planar bone scintigraphy, SPECT has been shown to be very advantageous in handling hard to reach places such as the anterior spine, temporomandibular joints (TMJs), internal regions of the skull, internal portions of the knees, and the accetabulum/femoral head regions of the pelvis and femurs. As with liver SPECT, the technical details are not complicated, nor timeconsuming. A number of institutions employ lumbar spine SPECT as a routine part of a bone scan, when the referral is made because of lower back pain.

Prior to data acquisition, proper COR and uniformity correction should be instituted. Acquisition of the skull may employ a

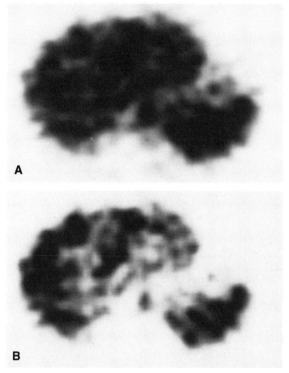

FIG. 10-3. Transaxial slice of a ^{99m}Tc-labeled RBC liver study with the application of (**A**) attenuation correction and (**B**) without attenuation correction. Note the increased liver edge activity when attenuation correction is not applied.

low-energy, all-purpose collimator, or an inverted slant-hole collimator as described in Chapter 4. Positioning and computer parameters are established in the same manner as decribed for brain perfusion studies. Collection of 64 frames at 25–30 sec per frame, onto a 64 × 64 matrix will yield suficient counts for diagnostic reconstruction. A low band-pass per filter such as Hann or Hamm with a 0.4 to 0.55 cutoff frequency will provide relatively smooth, but not too smooth, transaxial images that may be reorientated with sagittal/coronal software, or should patient positioning be a problem, the oblique reorientation software described in both Chapter 8 and 9 (Fig. 10–4).

Acquisition of the lumbar or thoracic spine will require the

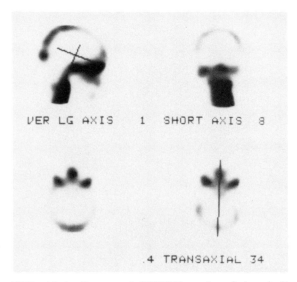

FIG. 10-4. Processed SPECT study of the skull demonstrating the utility of oblique reorientation software in situations where positioning may be less than optimal.

patient placing both arms above their head, and the detector rotating as close as possible to the body part required. The lumbar spine is an excellent target for which to employ an elliptical orbit acquisition technique, as the vast majority of lower back patients have abdomens of this shape. There are, naturally, very circular abdomens, and the technologist is left to his/her own devices and experience when setting up positional and collection criteria. The patient can be comforted a greate deal, regardless of condition, by elevating the knees with pillows, sponges, or stacks of sheets and blankets. This positioning also has the added benefit of bringing the lumbar spine somewhat closer to the table, and this to the detector in the posterior regions.

Reconstruction of the spine would again involve prefiltering the projection set with a low band-pass filter with a 0.04 to 0.6 rolloff. The user should be wary of excessive smoothing when reconstructing the spine. Ideally, the final images would be of such quality that the individual vertebral bodies could be distinguishable in the coronal views (Fig. 10–5A). Attempts to induce greater

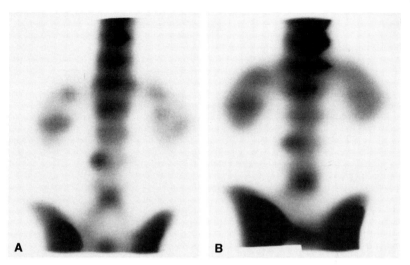

FIG. 10-5. (**A**) Coronal view of reconstructed lumbar spine SPECT demonstrating vertebral body separation. (**B**) Over filtering of the same study presenting a degraded image with resultant smearing of vertebral structures.

smoothing could degrade resolution enough to blurr each adjoining vertebral body into its neighbor (Fig. 10–5B).

The use of oblique reorientation software is again particularly helpful when dealing with bones that are not in a transaxial, coronal, or sagittal plane, such as the femoral head, or even at times the lumbar spine. The sagittal section of a lumbar spine (Fig. 10–6) demonstrates the curvature from posterior to anterior that could make separation of vertebral bodies difficult with standard transaxial slices. Reorientating these slices at user-selected angles may bring about a slightly altered set of transaxial and coronal slices that yield truer vertebra separation.

GALLIUM SPECT

The predominant soft-tissue, bone, and overall background activity of ^{67}Ga, presents an ideal situation for SPECT. Localization of absesses, certain tumor types, extent of *pneumocystis* pneumonia, and foci abnormal uptake in patients with Hodgkin's and non-Hodgkin's lymphoma has always been hampered by sur-

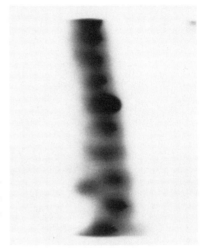

FIG. 10-6. Sagittal view of lumbar spine demonstrating the moderate curvature that may result in some structural overlapping in the transaxial plane.

rounding activity, giving gallium scintigraphy something of a bad name.

Gallium-67 scanning has played a controversial role in the management of patients with lymphoma, mostly because of false-negative results. However, these studies have included the use of low dose (3–5 mCi) ^{67}Ga and rectilinear scanners. More up-to-date studies with larger doses (up to 10 mCi), and triple-peak gamma cameras have reported standard planar imaging accuracy of 96%. Recent reports using SPECT as an additional technology, have demonstrated increased sensitivity from planar gallium imaging (0.66) to SPECT gallium imaging (0.96) in the chest, and 0.69 to 0.85 in the abdomen.

Previous studies with imaging gallium uptake in lymphoma had concentrated primarily on the detection of the disease. However, both the extent and the location of involvement must also be determined at the time of initial evaluation, as well as post-therapy follow-up. SPECT, because of its ability to separate different foci of abnormal uptake and to display images in transaxial, sagittal, and coronal planes, depicts the different abnormal nodal groups better than planar imaging. In addition, SPECT shows foci of disease not clearly demonstrated on some planar images.

In isolating an area of infection, SPECT has the advantage

of separating an abscess from surgical incisions, bowel, or nearby bone. In cases of dual problems, such as might be found in patients with AIDS, the gallium uptake of *pneumocystis* pneumonia (PCP) may over shadow the characteristic nodal uptake of lymphoma. SPECT is capable of distinguishing the diffuse pattern of the inflammatory process from the discrete foci chain of disease nodes, giving the clinician a better handle on the status of the disease.

Gallium-67 presents some technical problems not unlike those described in the chapter on brain perfusion SPECT with the ^{123}I compounds. Radionuclides with multiple-energy peaks, such as ^{67}Ga or ^{111}In, collected with dual or triple windows tend to produce some significant background scatter that is amplified in the reconstruction process.

Because it is the role of the Ramp filter to control low frequency background, the innovative alterations of the low or high bandpass windows are not quite as effective as one would like to see. For example, the low frequency scatter of the 186-keV photo peak of ^{67}Ga is theoretically supressed by the Ramp filter as well as the scatter of the 94-keV peak. Thus, the role of reducing the effects of multiple, amplified scatter from two or three photo peaks becomes a matter for those factors outside the reconstruction process to handle. The two most influential factors that immediately should come to mind are the collimator and pulse-height analyzers.

As with any part of the SPECT field, the choice of collimator is primarily one of living with what came with the system. However, if a technologist should find that, all factors being equal, the cross-sectional images of one system lack the contrast demonstrated by another, then the specifications of the collimator should be investigated. If the bore length is less than one might find on another brand, then this alone could be the cause of reduced contrast. The longer the length of the septa, the greater the absorbing potential and probability of absorption of secondary scatter from nonparallel primary photons. And, of course, with the higher energy photons that are characteristic of ^{67}Ga, the greater the probability that some form of secondary photon will be created from intertaction with the collimator septa. Therefore, the longer bore length will lower the chances of a given secondary photon reaching the crystal face.

Septal thickness is also a collimator characteristic that should be taken into account. Septal thickness combined with bore length may make a great difference in the degree of contrast present in a cross-sectional image, long before the reconstruction process.

The second device that should not be taken for granted is the window settings of the three pulse-height analyzers. Setting any one, or all three of the windows to greater widths to collect more counts only adds to degrade the final product. The windows should be tight enough to let in only the purest of photons, but at the same time provide enough counts for a statistically adequate study. A 20%, centered window about the three first photo peaks of ^{67}Ga will do. If, however, contrast of the reconstructed image is still less than desired, an asymetric 20% window might be tried, with the idea that a greater portion of compton scatter is removed prior to reconstruction.

The low statistics and even lower information density of a gallium study, even with a 10-mCi dose, tend to leave little choice in the selection of a reconstruction filter/window combination. A low band-pass filter such as a Hamm or Hann is recommended for prefiltering the projection set, with a straight Ramp applied during reconstruction. Because the statistical noise of ^{67}Ga SPECT is so great, the application of low-filter rolloffs will probably seem correct for first time attempts. The user can iterate through a number of filters and rolloffs (Fig. 10–7), but beware of inadequate smoothing. Too little smoothing, resulting in sharp, grainy images may mask discrete hot lesions as much or more than oversmoothing (Fig. 10–7D).

While imaged regions of gallium-avid foci are markedly improved with SPECT, two areas of concern have required further attention. In regions of the chest, only the sternum and spine provide reasonable anatomic landmarks for localizing gallium-avid foci, and this is usually restricted to the sagittal planes. Areas of increased uptake are not always readily placed within the chain of nodes following a path down the sides of the spine. Absolute placement of a "hot" spot is difficult at best, and usually a function of the interpreter's experience. In the abdomen, the left lobe of the liver may overwhelm gallium-avid nodes with less activity. In both circumstances, a technique is available that is not difficult

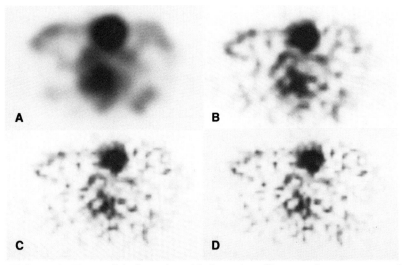

FIG. 10-7. Transaxial view of a mid-thoracic gallium study reconstructed with a Ramp-Hann filter at rolloffs of (**A**) 0.25, (**B**) 0.5, (**C**) 0.75, and (**D**) 1.00. Note that the areas of increased gallium activity in the sternum and spine become camouflaged with noise as the frequency cutoff is increased.

to perform, and requires little additional time.

If a patient is referred for gallium SPECT to evaluate or search for avid abdominal lymph nodes, a series of standard anterior and posterior high-resolution planar images may be followed by a 30-min SPECT study. Collected on a 64 × 64 matrix, for 30 sec per frame, totaling 64 frames in a 360-degree arc, the projection set is quickly reconstructed into transaxial images prior to the patient's dismissal. If these images present any questionable areas of increase activity in the region of the left lobe of the liver (Fig. 10-8), the patient may be injected with 3–5 mCi of ^{99m}Tc sulfur colloid, and reimaged with a ^{99m}Tc window, for 5–10 sec per frame for 64 frames. When collection is completed, and the patient released, both the gallium projection set and the ^{99m}Tc set are corrected for uniformity and stored. The mean counts of the liver in both sets are extrapolated, with the higher of the two reduced to the same mean as the lower, using image arithmetic software. This subtracted projection set is then prefiltered and reconstructed, presenting transaxial images that concentrate on the para aortic

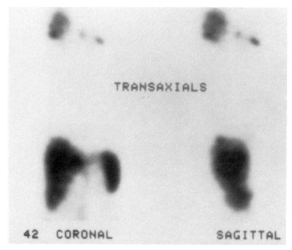

FIG. 10-8. Transaxial, coronal, and sagittal slices of an abdominal gallium study, presenting a questionable area of increased activity in the right upper lobe of the liver.

nodes surrounding the spine, in effect negating the influence of the liver (Fig. 10-9).

This same subtraction technique may be empoyed with the chest, using ^{99m}Tc-macroaggregated albumin (MAA) as the negating device. In cases of PCP overlapping or masking nodal activity due to lymphoma, the diffuse uptake of PCP is subtracted with the ^{99m}Tc-MAA and in effect enhancing the nodal activity. In addition, regions of increased activity in the chest, that are not nodal in origin, are anatomically better defined when a negative map of lung perfusion is overlayed. In both the chest and abdomen, the trick to the technique is to be sure the patient has not moved the target area during the time between acquisitions. Again, either of these processes add only 8–10 min to the patient's acquisition time.

The use of ^{67}Ga scintigraphy is increasing in many clinics for a number of reasons: it is inexpensive; it can achieve high sensitivity and accuracy; it is not an investigational tool requiring a great deal of oversight; and current instruments are a substantial improvement over those that attempted gallium imaging in the

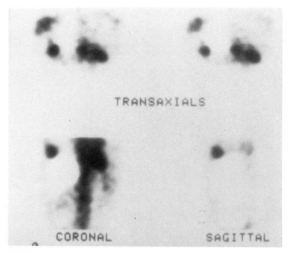

FIG. 10-9. Transaxial, coronal, and sagittal slices after subtraction of a ^{99m}Tc-sulfur colloid liver SPECT from the gallium SPECT. Gallium-avid foci on the right upper lobe of the liver presents itself posteriorly and above the diaphragm.

past. As with other radiopharmaceuticals, SPECT provides a new dimension and potential to gallium scintigraphy.

SUGGESTED READINGS

1. Turner DA, Fordam EW, Ali A, et al. Gallium-67 imaging in management of Hodgkin's disease and other malignant lymphoma. *Semin Nucl Med* 1978;8:205–218.

2. Johnston GS, Go MF, Benua RS, et al. Gallium-67 citrate imaging in Hodgkin's disease: Final report of a cooperative group. *J Nucl Med* 1977;18:692–698.

3. Andrews GA, Hubner KF, Greenlaw RH. Gallium-67 citrate imaging in malignant lymphoma: Final report of a cooperative group. *J Nucl Med* 1978;19:1013–1019.

4. Anderson KC, Leonard RCF, Canellos CP, et al. High dose gallium in lymphoma. *Am J Med* 1983;75:327–331.

5. Hoffer PB, Schor R, Ashby D, et al. Comparison of Ga-67 images obtained with rectilinear scanner in large field Anger camera. *J Nucl Med* 1977;18:538–540.

ANSWERS TO STUDY QUESTIONS

Chapter 2	Chapter 3	Chapter 4	Chapter 5	Chapter 6
1. e	1. e	1. e	1. a	1. f
2. d	2. d	2. b	2. e	2. f
3. b	3. f	3. b	3. f	3. f
4. e	4. f	4. d	4. d	4. e
5. f	5. f	5. c	5. b	5. b
6. e	6. e	6. c	6. f	6. e
7. c	7. e	7. f	7. e	7. d
8. c	8. f	8. f		8. e
	9. f	9. c		9. e
	10. f	10. c		10. b
		11. f		11. f
				12. f
				13. c
				14. f

APPENDIX

APPENDIX A
Quality-Control Suggestions

DAILY

Uniformity analysis
  5-million-count field flood—uncorrected
  5-million-count field flood—corrected

Energy spectrum analysis

Collimator integrity (visual inspection)

WEEKLY

30-million-count flood collection—extrinsic
  (with applicable radionuclide if necessary)

Center-of-rotation acquisition and analysis
  (with each collimator utilized)

Table/detector alignment

Detector/collection matrix alignment

MONTHLY

Pixel sizing

Intrinsic and extrinsic FWHM/FWTM

QUARTERLY

Acquisition of cylindrical SPECT phantom

Analyzed uniformity resolution (hot and cold)

APPENDIX B
SPECT Data-Collection Examples

Study	Isotope	Dose (mCi)	Time Delay	Collimator	Number of Projections	Matrix Size	Seconds per Projection	Magnification Factor	Disk Utilization	Window Consideration
Bone	99mTc-DP	20	3 hr	LEAP, GAP	60–64	64 × 64	20–25	1.0	1,025 blocks	Single peak
Brain	99mTc-GH	20	3 hr	LEAP, GAP	60–64	64 × 64	30–40	1.5	1,025 blocks	Single peak
Brain	123I-amine	5	20 min	LEAP, SLANT Long-bore	60–64	64 × 64	30–40	1.0	1,025 blocks	Single peak
Liver	99mTc-sulfur colloid	3	20 min	LEAP, GAP	60–64	64 × 64	20–25	1.0	1,025 blocks	Single peak
				HR	120–128	128 × 128	20–25	1.0	8,200 blocks	Single peak
				LEAP, GAP	120–128	64 × 64	10–12	1.0	2,050 blocks	Single peak
Liver	99mTc-RBC	20	1–2 hr	LEAP, GAP	60–64	64 × 64	20–25	1.0	1,025 blocks	Single peak
Gallium	67Ga-citrate	5–10	48–72 hr	Medium energy	60–64	64 × 64	30–40	1.0	1,025 blocks	Triple peak
Myocardial	201Tl-chloride	2	Immediate post- and 2–4 hr postexercise	LEAP, GAP	32/180°	64 × 64	40	1.0	513 blocks	Dual peak
					64/180°	64 × 64	20	1.0	1,025 blocks	Dual peak
					64/360°	64 × 64	40	1.0	1,025 blocks	Dual peak
					128/360°	64 × 64	20	1.0	2,050 blocks	Dual peak

APPENDIX C
SPECT Overview

QUALITY CONTROL

Standard gamma camera quality
    control
Uniformity correction
Center of rotation

ACQUISITION

Continuous versus step and shoot
Matrix selection
Collection time
Number of projections
$360°$ versus $180°$
Collimator selection
Uniformity correction and attenuation
    correction on the fly (yes or no)

PROCESSING

Uniformity correction
Prefiltering
Transaxial reconstruction
Number of slices
Slice thickness
Reconstruction filter cutoff attenuation
    parameters

DISPLAY

Sagittal, coronal, oblique
Slice thickness
Plane orientation selection
Final display format

APPENDIX D
Mathematical Model of Backprojection

Using the x,y coordinate system shown in Figure D-1 as a representation of a source's cross-sectional distribution, the detector at angle Θ would collect counts from each pixel $f(x,y)$ along projection path t as a total sum. If $f(x,y)$ is the value of radioactivity at point (x,y), t could be defined as

$$t = [x\cos(\Theta) + y\sin(\Theta)].$$

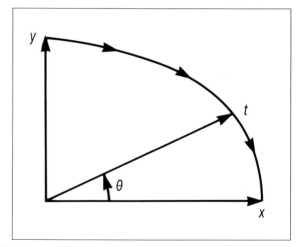

FIG. D-1. Acquisition path of the rotating gamma camera plotted on an x,y coordinate system. (Courtesy of Nahmias C, Kenyon DB, Kouris K, et al, *Single Photon Emission Computed Tomography and Other Selected Computer Topics.* The Society of Nuclear Medicine, 1980:20.)

If the function $p(t, \Theta)$ represents the projected data, or the total sum of activity along the line integral t at angle Θ, then

$$p(t, \Theta) = \int f(x,y)\delta(x\cos\Theta + y\sin\Theta - t)d_x d_y$$

with the delta function δ restricting the line integral to the line $t = x\cos\Theta + y\sin\Theta$.

The simplest method of reconstruction is to assign $p(t, \Theta)$ back onto the reconstruction plane, so that $p(t, \Theta)$ is assigned to each picture element (pixel) along the path of (t, Θ), the acquisition path, yielding

$$f(x,y) = \int_0^\pi p(t\Theta)d_\Theta.$$

The integral symbols represent the summed data along each projection p, from Θ to π, or the complete $360°$ arc.

As this model demonstrates, the points on the reconstruction plane that overlap generate an addition process of $f(x,y)$ and therefore a localization of that region from a different perspective. However, the problem of assigning $f(x,y)$ to each pixel along the angled path creates a "star" effect.

APPENDIX E
Mathematics of Filters/Windows Used in SPECT Reconstruction

Convolution filtering is the most popular method of filtered back-projection. This technique can be demonstrated with a solution similar to that obtained from two-dimensional Fourier reconstruction (Appendix F) if a backprojected ray sum is modified. If simple backprojection is demonstrated as

$$f_{bp}(x,y) \; = \; p(t,\Theta)d_\Theta,$$

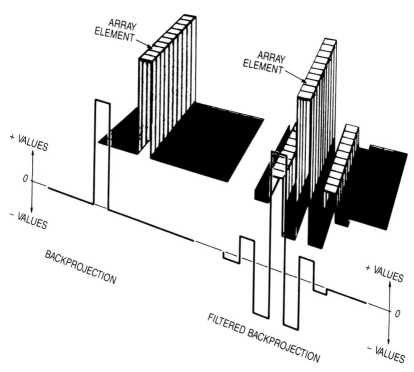

FIG. E-1. Filtered backprojection. In the backprojection method (left), the value assigned to an array element is the complete ray sum, with no effort made to correct for nontarget activity (i.e., background, noise) resulting in the criss-cross of nontarget activity and resultant "star" effect. In filtered backprojection (right), the negative value assigned to each side of the ray sum affects the neighboring array element, thereby reducing "star" effects. (Courtesy of Brooks RA, DiChiro G, *Phys Med Biol* 1976;21(5):689–732.)

then a density histogram might be plotted as shown in Figure E-1. The composite of all the angulated projections will yield a "star" artifact. This backprojection technique can be related to the two-dimensional Fourier transform by the introduction of a filter factor $|K|$:

$$|K| \; F_{bp}(k_x, k_y) \;=\; P(k, \Theta) \;=\; F(k_x, k_y).$$

Basically, the higher-frequency components of the projected data are amplified by a factor equal to the absolute value of the frequency $|K|$. In essence, if it is accepted that useful data are in the lower frequency range, and noise is in the higher, then the frequency factor $|K|$ can be altered to extract only the information desired. The resultant plot of this technique may appear as that shown in Figure E-1.

As described previously in this text, the Ramp filter is the basic reconstruction function that removes the "star" artifact inherent in the reconstruction process. This filter and its associated window functions are best described in frequency space, or more simply put, the filter function plotted as a function of the cycles per pixel, which will be termed kx in the following examples. Because the Ramp filter is simply a straight line, it may be generated easily by plotting kx as a function of kx. Should an additional filter be incorporated with the Ramp filter, then its mathematical expression is simply multiplied by kx and plotted as a function of kx. For example, a filter function whose expression is $\cos(kx/kx \bullet m)$ would be simply be combined with the Ramp filter to form the expression $x \bullet [\cos(kx/kx \bullet m)]$. Outlined below are some of the more common filters, their relationship with the Ramp filter, and, the resultant plots. For simplicity, we will use only one-dimensional functions (i.e., functions of the single variable of spatial frequency kx or the frequency in the x direction.) In reality, the filters are often two-dimensional functions, depending on frequency in the y direction, ky.

Ramp Filter Without a Window Function

$kx = 0,0.1..1$ where $f(kx) = x.$

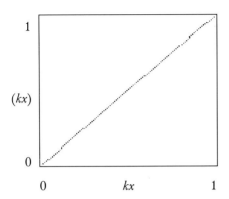

Shepp and Logan Without the Ramp Filter

$kx = 0,0.1..1$

$$SL(kx) = \frac{sin(kx)}{kx}$$

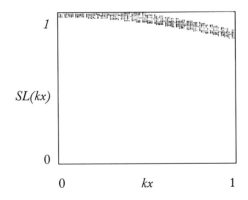

Ramp with Shepp and Logan

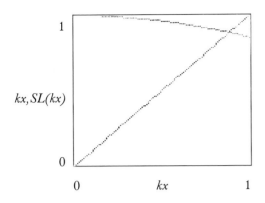

Ramp Filter when Multiplied to the Shepp and Logan

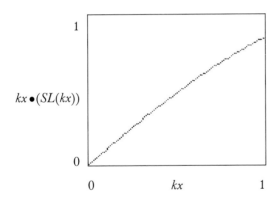

Hamming and Hann Filters with the Ramp Filter

Cutoff frequency: $xm = 0.5$,

where cutoff frequency is a user-defined frequency in which data in the image approaches zero. (If, for example, a 64×64 matrix was employed, the maximum number of cycles would be 32/64, or 0.5. Therefore, a cutoff >0.5 would result in a mirror effect, or alliasing.)

$$\text{Ham}(x) = 0.54 + 0.46 \times \cos\left[\pi \frac{x}{xm}\right]$$

$$\text{Ham}(kx) = 0.5 + 0.5 \times \cos\left[\pi \frac{kx}{xm}\right]$$

kx is defined as 0 at frequencies greater than xm.

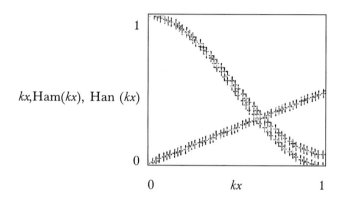

Ramp Filter Multiplied to the Hann Window

In this function, the standard Ramp-Hann filter is formed with a frequency cutoff of 0.5.

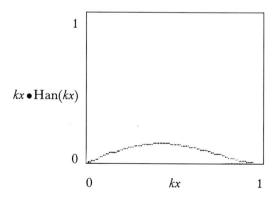

Butterworth Filter with a Ramp Filter Overlay

Power is n, $n = 5$.
$xm = 0.5$

$$\text{But}\,(kx) = \frac{1}{1 + \left[\dfrac{kx}{xm}\right]^{2 \bullet n}}$$

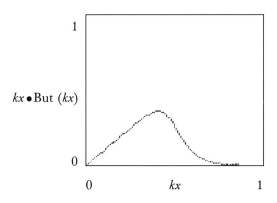

kx, But (kx) vs kx (axes from 0 to 1)

Ramp Filter Multiplied to the Butterworth Filter

This function demonstrates a steeper descending slope than the Ramp-Hann filter window.

$kx \bullet \text{But}\,(kx)$ vs kx (axes from 0 to 1)

APPENDIX F
Two-Dimensional Fourier Transformation

A flexible tool for filter characterization and image reconstruction is the Fourier transform, a mathematical process that decomposes a data-set waveform into more fundamental waveforms. For example, a profile of an image, or better still the x row of pixels, may be broken down into components representing the relative contribution of low, middle, and high spatial frequencies. Thus, for image reconstruction, a conversion of the radionuclide distribution and resultant density, $f(x,y)$, from real to frequency domain, could be expressed as the Fourier integral:

$$f(x,y) = \int\int F(k_x,k_y)\exp 2\pi i(k_x x + k_y y)\, dk_x dk_y.$$

This Fourier integral may be dissected to make some sense if one considers $f(x,y)$ the density or counts of a pixel to be unknown. Points kx, ky represent spatial frequency in the x and y directions and the notation $\exp[2\pi i]$ represents an alternative method of expressing $\cos\Theta + i\sin\Theta$. The integral symbols represent a summing or totaling procedure and $F(k_x,k_y)$ the Fourier coefficients that may be obtained using an inverse Fourier transform:

$$F(k_x,k_y) = \int\int f(x,y)\exp[-2\pi i(k_x x + k_y y)]d_x d_y.$$

As has been described earlier, the radionuclide density to be determined, $f(x,y)$, and the ray sum measured $p(t,\Theta)$ are related:

$$p(t,\Theta) = \int f(x,y)\, \delta\, (x\cos\Theta + y\sin\Theta - t)d_x d_y.$$

It can be mathematically determined that $F(k_x,k_y)$ is equal to $p(k,\Theta)$, and $p(k,\Theta)$ is the Fourier transform of $p(t,\Theta)$. This projection equation is fundamental for analytic reconstruction, since it relates the Fourier transform of a known quantity $p(t\Theta)$ (that measured by a detector) to the Fourier transform of the sought-after unknown function $f(x,y)$.

The two-dimensional Fourier transform technique can then be stated in four basic steps:

1. Measure all the ray sums, $p(t,\Theta)$.
2. Calculate the Fourier transform of the ray sums, $p(k,\Theta)$.
3. This transform is equal to the two-dimensional transform of the density distribution.
4. An inverse Fourier transform is performed to yield $f(x,y)$.

APPENDIX G
Concepts of Attenuation Correction

Several first-order correction methods have been proposed to compensate for attenuation. One precorrection approach, from Sorenson, is known as the hyperbolic sine correction to the geometric mean of opposing projections (Fig. G-1). Assume that the activity is distributed uniformly within a larger absorbing medium of constant attenuation u. Also assume that a measured projection ray traverses a distance L of absorber along which the fractional length fL has a constant source strength C. For this simplified case, it can be shown that a corrected projection measurement at angle Θ and lateral position x is given by

$$p_{corr}(x,\Theta) = p'_{gcom}(x,\Theta) \cdot ufl \cdot e^{ufl/2}/(2\sinh(ufl/2)),$$

where $p'_{gcom}(x,\Theta)$ is the geometric (or conjugate) mean of opposing projections (the square root of the product of opposing line integral measurements).

Rather than using the geometric mean, Kay and Keys proposed using the arithmetic mean (average) of opposing projections. For this case, their corrected projection was

$$p_{corr}(x,\Theta) = 4p'_{arith}(x,\Theta)/(1 + e^{-ul} + 2e^{-ul/2}).$$

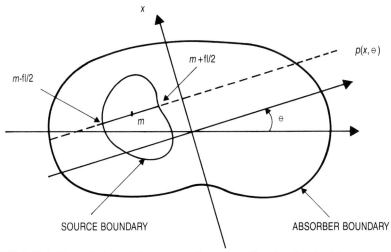

FIG. G-1. Knowledge of the extent of a source distribution inside attenuating material can be used to help compensate for attenuation. (Courtesy of Moore SC, *Computed Emission Tomography.* Oxford University Press.)

A simple postcorrection method was proposed by Chang. After reconstructing an image without any attenuation correction, each pixel in the image is multiplied by the following correction factor:

$$C(x,y) = \left[\frac{1}{m}\sum_{i=1}^{m}\exp(-ul(x,y,\Theta_i))\right]^{-1},$$

where $l(x,y)$ is the distance from the point (x,y) to the boundary of the attenuating material along the projection ray at the angle perpendicular to the detector and traverses the point (x,y). Thus, the correction factor is the inverse of the averaged measured attenuation of a source at the point (x,y). If the true distribution of attenuating material is known, this correction factor could be modified by integrating this distribution along the lines $l(x,y,\Theta)$.

The reconstructed SPECT image will not be accurate for all possible distributions of source and attenuating material using these first-order methods. Simple multiplicative corrections cannot resolve the SPECT measurement ambiguity described earlier. Other more elaborate methods, such as an analytic method for convex uniform attenuators (Tretiak and Gullberg, see Chapter 2 Suggested Readings), or several iterative techniques, can often provide more accurate results but usually require longer computing times.

One iterative method, developed by Moore et al. for a multidetector SPECT scanner, has recently been used successfully for a rotating gamma camera system (Faber, see Chapter 2 Reading List). The steps in this technique are as follows:

1. Reconstruct a starting image, $f(x,y)$, using a "standard" (filtered backprojection) technique, corrected to first order for attenuation using the Chang method previously described.
2. Estimate the projection data that would be seen if scanning this image estimate.
3. Subtract each estimated projection from the corresponding real measured projection data to form error projections.
4. Reconstruct the error projections to form an error image, $\Delta^i(x,y)$ for the ith iteration.
5. Use the error image to calculate a damping factor 6^i, which minimizes χ^2 (chi-square).
6. Obtain the next image by calculating:

$$f^{i+1}(x,y) = f^i(x,y) + 6^i \bullet \Delta^i(x,y)$$

for all pixels (x,y).

7. Go to step 2 and repeat until the estimated projection data match the real data within the statistical errors (minimum χ^2).

Other iterative methods are similar to this one. The way in which they often differ from one another is a function of how the error projections are used to correct the image of each iteration. One advantage to iterative methods is that they can use an "exact" attenuation distribution (such as from a CT scan of the same cross section) instead of simple ellipsoidal shapes with the assumption of uniform attenuation inside the ellipses.

GLOSSARY

ADC (analog-to-digital converter): An electronic component that alters voltage gradients from the gamma camera into binary data required by the computer.

Algorithm: Computer instructions, in higher- or lower-level software, that step the computer through its functions.

Amines: Analogs of naturally occurring compounds that act as chemical mediators of brain function. When labeled with ^{123}I, amines are used in brain-perfusion studies.

Amplitude: The increments on the y axis of data plotted in frequency space; the y limit in the filtering process.

Analog: Signals that have multiple gradients; voltages that originate from the gamma camera are of varying intensities, usually proportional to the detected event, and are thus analog.

Analytic reconstruction: A set of reconstruction algorithms that have a single unique solution, i.e., the Fourier and convolution reconstruction algorithms.

Arc: A portion or section of a 360-degree circumference.

ART (algebraic reconstruction technique): A type of iterative algorithm for reconstruction that begins with the first projection being backprojected. Each progressive projection is then compared with a projection made from the reconstruction matrix. A derived projection is backprojected and the cycle is repeated throughout the entire set of projections. (See Iterative)

Artifacts: Those portions of an image that do not exist in the original source; they may be due to background, noise, patient movement, or instrument malfunction.

Attenuation: The absorption of a photon, or charged particle, by matter.

Attenuation correction: Mathematical methods of compensating for photon absorption as a function of target-to-detector distance.

Backprojection: The additive, Moire, or summation techniques of image reconstruction from projections; the simplest but least precise method of image reconstruction.

Bull's-eye artifact: A circular nonuniformity in a reconstructed image. An artifact with its primary cause originating from poor or improper uniformity correction.

Butterworth filter: A smoothing window with an adjustable bandwidth.

Center of rotation: A quality-control procedure that establishes the best possible projection-to-projection relationship in a detector's rotational orbit, and corrects for discrepancies.

Chang attenuation correction: An iterative procedure. A first-order correction is performed and reprojected; reprojections are then compared with measured projections, and error projections are backprojected to form an error image, which is added to first order.

Circular orbit: A scintillation detector's mode of acquisition travel during tomographic studies; often a source of target-to-detector distance problems with noncircular sources.

Continuous rotation: A nonstop method of photon acquisition during tomographic data collection; data collected during this nonstop process are reformatted into discrete angle-related frames or projections.

Contrast: A system's ability to distinguish objects of varying sizes or colors from its surrounding activity.

Convolution filtering: The mathematical technique used in filtered backprojection; the method of applying a negative value to both sides of the density histogram of each ray sum before the final backprojection.

COR (center of rotation): The camera's axis of rotation. (See Center of rotation)

Coronal tomographic sections: Those sections that are at right angles to the transverse sections, usually from anterior to posterior.

Cucumber slices: Reoriented oblique slices that follow a line from the base of the left ventricle to the apex.

DCAT (dynamic computer-assisted tomography): An early SPECT instrument developed by Stokely to image dynamic studies tomographically.

Digital: Extrapolation of analog signals that exist in only one of two states, on or off, with no intermediate level between these two states; the necessary form that scintillation signals must possess for computer manipulation.

ECT: See Emission computed tomography.

Elliptical orbit: The scintillation detector's mode of travel during the SPECT acquisition process that follows a path closer to the patient's body contour.

Emission computed tomography (ECT): The cross-sectional reconstruction imaging of single-photon or positron radiopharmaceuticals and agents.

Filtered backprojection: Reconstruction algorithms that mathematically attempt to remove or suppress nontarget data before backprojection.

Filters: Mathematical operations designed to enhance, smooth, or suppress part or all of digital-image data.

Fourier analysis: The method of analyzing shapes in terms of their individual frequency waveforms; the Fourier transform is the determination of sine and cosine waves to synthesize a shape.

Frequency: The occurrence of an incident or waveform per unit time or distance; the maximum frequency for 64 pixels is 32.

Frequency cutoff: That point of an image's frequency characteristics that is accepted for image reconstruction; the higher the frequency, the noisier the image; the lower-frequency cutoffs provide for smoother images.

Fourier transformation: The mathematical technique of converting the repetitions of a situation into sine or cosine functions.

FWHM (full width at half maximum): A measurement of line spread function that will provide information on collimator resolution. FWHM is the distance between the two points where the count rate falls off to 50% on the focal plane where the count rate is 100%.

FWTM (full width at tenth maximum): The distance between two points where the count rate falls off to 10% on the focal plane where the count rate is 100%. (See FWHM)

Hamming: A smoothing window with an adjustable frequency cutoff.

Hann: A smoothing window with an adjustable frequency cutoff. A common, commercially available two-dimensional window.

Intrinsic spatial resolution: The best possible separation of two line sources at the face of the crystal (collimator off).

ILST (iterative least squares technique): A type of iterative algorithm for reconstruction. (See Iterative)

Iterative: The repetitive mathematical calculation of a problem, beginning with the best-guess estimate, until the resolution of the problem to the closest possible result.

Linearity: The amount of positional distortion caused by the camera with respect to incident gamma events entering the detector.

Matrix: The x,y array of pixels and/or memory elements provided by the computer for storage or display. Basically a square with equal x,y divisions.

MRI (magnetic resonance imaging): A modality that provides high contrast cross-sectional images without ionizing radiation. The principle involves the measuring of emitted radio signals from atomic nuclei placed in a strong magnetic field stimulated by a radiofrequency.

Necrosis: Decay or death of tissue as a result of loss of blood supply.

NEMA (National Electrical Manufacturers Association): An organization of manufacturers who develop specifications and guidelines for the minimal acceptable standards for equipment.

Noise: Unwanted contributions to an image from background and/or scatter radiation or as statistical fluctuations in measurements.

Nyquist frequency: That point at which a filter's transfer function begins to fold or become a mirror of itself.

Partial volume effect: The overlap of counts experienced between two adjoining slices; the number two slice in a three-slice study would contain a portion of counts from the first and third slices.

PET: See Positron emission tomography.

Pixel: Those elements of an image matrix that are the individual location counts; short for picture element.

Planar projections: The individual static images, acquired at a set predefined orientation.

Poisson: A principle that states that the standard deviation is proportional to the square root of the number of observed events.

Positron: A particle having a mass equal to the electron and having an equal but opposite charge; production of positrons yields two oppositely directed 511-keV gamma photons.

Positron emission tomography (PET): Cross-sectional images of positron radionuclide distribution.

Projections: The planar or static images collected at predefined angles around a target that provide the raw data for a reconstructed image.

PTCA (Percutaneous transluminal coronary angioplasty): A nonsurgical procedure for relieving regional myocardial ischemia caused by coronary artery disease. This invasive technique will dilate the arterial lumen by inflating a balloon catheter thereby permitting improved blood flow.

Quantitation: A numerical description of radiotracer localization within a physiologic region.

Ramp filter: A linear filter function that suppresses adjacent overlying pixel activity. The most common commercial filter used in filtered backprojection.

Rolloffs: The frequency point at which a window reaches cutoff.

Sagittal sections: Slices perpendicular to the transverse plane that cut lateral to medial.

SIRT (simultaneous iterative reconstruction technique): A type of iterative algorithm for reconstruction. (See Iterative)

Smoothing: Mathematical manipulation of data that reduces the sharp pixel-to-pixel, or frame-to-frame, count changes; a method of normalizing adjoining data while attempting to preserve detail.

Single-photon emission computed tomography: See ECT.

Star effect: The radiating arms of source data inherent in any type of backprojection; an artifact common to improper reconstruction filters, inadequate numbers of projections, and/or irregularities in the rotational field of view.

Step and shoot: An acquisition technique that collects independent planar angulated projections before filtered backprojection; the prereconstruction raw data are a set number of complete static frame-mode images.

Tomography: From the Greek words "to cut or section" (tomos) and "to write" (graphein); a method of separating overlying and underlying interference from the source or target of interest by imaging a cut section of the object.

Transverse sections: The horizontal slices at right angles to the vertical axis of the body; the initial tomographic images acquired and used for reconstruction; those images perpendicular to the axis of detector rotation.

Uniformity: The count distribution across the field of view of a scintillation gamma camera.

Voxel: Three-dimensional picture elements; in a three-slice study, each pixel in the middle slice attains a third dimension of depth from the adjoining first- and third-slice pixels; short for volume element.

Window: The mathematical function in frequency space that controls the filter's acceptance of data; that portion of the filter that may be altered or designed to accept or suppress certain components of data as desired.

INDEX

NOTES

NOTES

NOTES

NOTES